D0457443

YOU DON'T KNOW
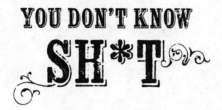

"By Patience, minds an equal temper know,
Nor swell too high, nor sink too low;
Patience the fiercest grief can charm,
And fate's severest rage disarm;
Patience can soften pain to ease,
And make despair and madness please;
This the divine Cecilia found,
And to her Husbands ears, confin'd the sound."

Pub.d Sept.r 19th 1791. by H. Humphrey. N.18. Old Bond Street

Vide St Cecilia's Day

"PATIENCE on a MONUMENT."

Engraved from a Modern Antique, in the possession of the General.

YOU DON'T KNOW
SH*T

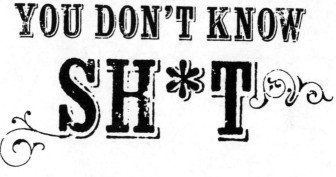

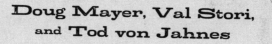

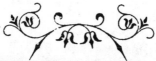

Doug Mayer, Val Stori, and Tod von Jahnes

ST. MARTIN'S GRIFFIN ❧ NEW YORK

YOU DON'T KNOW SH*T. Copyright © 2011 by Doug Mayer, Val Stori, and Tod von Jahnes. All rights reserved. Printed in the United States of America. For information, address St. Martin's Press, 175 Fifth Avenue, New York, N.Y. 10010.

www.stmartins.com

Designed by Ralph Fowler/rlfdesign

Library of Congress Cataloging-in-Publication Data

Mayer, Doug.
    You don't know sh*t / Doug Mayer, Val Stori, and Tod von Jahnes.—1st ed.
        p. cm.
    ISBN 978-0-312-64990-6
    1. Defecation—Social aspects.   2. Feces.   3. Flatulence.
I. Stori, Valerie.   II. Von Jahnes, Tod.   III. Title.   IV. Title: You don't know shit.   V. Title: You do not know shit.
    GT2835.M39 2011
    394—dc23

                                                                2011020533

ISBN 978-1-250-17259-4 (Special Edition)

Our books may be purchased in bulk for promotional, educational, or business use. Please contact your local bookseller or the Macmillan Corporate and Premium Sales Department at 1-800-221-7945, extension 5442, or by email at MacmillanSpecialMarkets@macmillan.com.

First Special Edition: October 2017

10 9 8 7 6 5 4 3 2 1

Contents

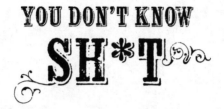

YOU DON'T KNOW
SH*T

BOTTOMS UP

Inter faeces et urinam nascimur!

We are born amid feces and urine," declaimed Saint Bernard of Clairvaux in the Middle Ages— a sermon that effectively kicked off one thousand years of general apprehension toward all things shit.

It didn't have to be that way. While we can thank our innermost reptile brains for keeping us from playing with what emerges from our derrieres, the fact is, most of our disgust over dropping trou is the result of what university types would term cultural socialization. In other words, what your mom told you, what Mr. Whipple told your mom, and so on—right back to that lousy lecture by Saint Bernard.

As any school nurse could tell you, shitting is a basic bodily function and a nice poop (which would earn a score of 4 on the Bristol stool scale—more on that later) is important for good health. If you're unsure, just look into the desperate eyes of anyone who hasn't pooped in a week. But how we poop, where we poop, and how we treat that poop? Well, that's all in our hands, in a manner of speaking.

All of which makes looking at the world through shit-colored lenses very interesting. Why? Because, you can tell a shitload about people by the way they poop, the changes in how they poop, and a comparison of their shit with—you're getting the hang of this now—other people's shit. Not that we're asking you to do all that, mind you. That's our job. And the results, from the space shuttle to the Serengeti, are in the pages that follow.

Why Shit Matters

The need to take a crap is universal. To shit is to be. And to be . . . well, that requires a little bit of thought. As in, "How am I going to act if my nosy neighbor looks in through the blinds and catches me wiping my ass?" What shitting means to our dignity has changed over the years, too. Romans didn't give a poop: they shat cheerily alongside a dozen fellow citizens, each also in mid-droppage. But when medieval monks started shitting alone, everything changed. Suddenly we couldn't poop without thinking about privacy. "Will anyone hear me? How can I mask the noise my ass is about to make? Why did I have to see Mom taking a dump?"

Shitting is also a timeless biological bond with our ancestors. When we shit, we're practically reaching out across the centuries and saying, "Hey, you, too?" Our poop is a common bond that no amount of flushing can wash asunder. Okay, maybe we're getting a bit carried away. But what else do we share almost identically with our knuckle-dragging ancestors? Not much. (At least for most of us.)

But once it's out of our asses, all bets are off. Whether we regard our poo as the embodiment of immoral filth, a colon-powered gold mine, or something in between is entirely up to us.

Or perhaps you're in touch with your inner Sigmund Freud and have come full circle, embracing your feces (though later in this book, we will admonish you to never touch your poo). Maybe you even see the act of pooping as a transformative, rejuvenating process.

Or you might view your shit as the ultimate recycling effort, culminating in valuable fertilizer and tasty tomatoes that have that certain je ne sais quoi.

Heck, you can even view your poop as a lucrative resource to be—pardon the image—mined. Chinese night soil? Of course! Money in the bank at the local fecal biogas station? Definitely! Night cream? It's been done. A drug you can ferment and huff? That, too, though we wish we hadn't reminded ourselves.

Shit matters for one other reason, too. Most notably because we still can't seem to get it under control. From the emptying of chamber pots onto medieval streets to the unabashed use of the Thames as an open sewer, shit in the wrong place continues to be the most basic sanitation problem that haunts our sorry asses. By now, you'd think we'd have our shit together.

Striking a Blow Against Fecal Invisibility

Here's a sad fact: Four million years after we stood upright and dropped our first load, humans can't speak openly about taking a crap. Only little kids remain unsullied by prudishness. Adults talk apologetically about "going to the comfort station" or "dropping the kids off at the pool." Taking a shit remains hidden and disguised—unless you've had a few beers too many and are asking your pals for the third time, "What's brown and sits on a piano?" (Answer: Beethoven's first movement.)

It's the same the world over. In developing countries, poopers scuttle about in low light, crouch among the bushes, and hurry through their business like it's all a bad dream. At the same time, in the "modern" world, we ensconce ourselves in sanitized cubicles, seated upon Japan's George Jetson–style Washlet, which goes so far as to make sounds to mask your own. Even the trusty American Standard is an enabler, making it easy for us to empty our colon, and—voilà!—with the push of a lever all evidence that we created a fecal monster is down the drain.

Well, we've had enough of fecal invisibility. We're pulling

back the shit-encrusted veil and taking a close, unembarrassed look at our dumps—whether it's onboard the space shuttle, a log floating down the Brahmaputra, or a thin veneer on your computer monitor. (It is. Sorry. More on that later.)

My Shit Is Your Shit

Now that we've dragged the brown beast out of the water closet, we can also sing shit's praises. Imagine if we could all talk about shit as freely as we liked. Maybe we'd actually be able to clean it up the world over?

And so, when you've finished with this shit-filled journey, we hope that the innermost part of your colon twinges with peristalsis, in recognition of your fellow poopers the planet over. Along the way, we hope you'll have gained a fresh perspective on the body's most basic function. Perhaps you'll even be inspired to spring for a new ultra-high-tech Toto Washlet . . . or hook up your toilet to your cookstove . . . or do something about your toothbrush, which, we have to tell you, lies within the fecal fallout zone. (It does. Sorry. More on that later.)

One thousand years after Saint Bernard started us down the wrong path, we think it's high time someone set the record straight and shouted to the world, *Ego defaeco, tu defaecas, nos omnes defaecamus. Quis nescit?* Or, in English, "I shit, you shit, we all shit. So what's the big deal?"

❧ 1 ❧

SHITTING THROUGH
THE AGES

The scent of artificial lilacs wafts through your bathroom. You rise from your sanitary porcelain throne, glance casually down (hey, it's okay—we all do), press a lever, and watch as your latest creation vanishes down the pipe.

But have you ever thought about what pooping must have been like long before the Ty-D-Bol Man, Mr. Whipple, and your local plumber helped make it all go *away*?

Imagine dropping trou alongside twenty neighbors. Or pinching a loaf as a humble offering to Sterculius, the Roman god of feces. Or entertaining guests while seated on your "throne," then having a "groom of the stool" wipe and possibly even kiss your ass? It all happened many poops ago.

And where did all that shit go, in the days of yore? We left it in our cave. We tossed it out the window and hollered, "Gardyloo!" Or we pooped into the moat—an unhappy surprise for attackers, but a thoughtful thank-you for the hungry fish far below.

As always, some cultures beat others to the pinch. Londoners were still heaving the contents of their chamber pots onto the streets dozens of centuries *after* the ancient Greeks had invented perfectly good sewage systems.

The history of shit is as rich and as varied as, well, poop itself. To take a look at where it first started, we first need to do a little digging. Literally.

Some Really Old Shit

Ancient civilizations have left all kinds of clues for archaeologists, from arrowheads to pottery shards. For some archaeologists, though, the Holy Grail isn't a golden chalice, but a petrified brown lump.

Why are fossilized feces such a field day for archaeologists? Find just one and you can figure out the gender of the dumper and his or her diet and diseases—even the bacteria and viruses that he or she might have been carrying around.

With all that information just a poop away, it's easy to imagine that a team of scientists digging in the Paisley 5 Mile Point Cave in Oregon must have high-fived each other when they found six piles of super-special shit that was really, *really* old.

The year was 2002, and the team had found the oldest shits ever discovered in the New World. And what did it look like after all those years? Said one team member, "Basically it looks like what it is: poop."

But what poops they were! Radiocarbon dating revealed the poops to be 12,300 RCYBP (radiocarbon years before the present)—meaning humans had been living in the Americas more than a thousand years earlier than previously thought. Not only that, but this shit had more in common with its Siberian relatives than with other poops in the Americas. Meaning the New World's earliest residents weren't actually natives. They dropped in after a long walk or a boat trip down the Alaskan coast.

As for their diet, those first Americans pooped out quite a range of morsels, including squirrel, bison, fish, birds, plants—even, we're loath to admit, a few dogs.

❧❦❧ DEEP SHIT!

Want to freshen up some old poo? Here's how archaeologist Dr. Eric Callen does it: Soak it in a solution of 0.5 percent trisodium phosphate for forty-eight hours, and bingo! Poop up to ten thousand years old is almost as good as new.

Who knew poo could be so telling? University of Oregon archaeologist Dennis Jenkins did. As one of the scientists who found the Paisley Cave shit, he said, "You don't think of it, but you're leaving behind genetic signatures every morning." (Another reason to double-check that everything goes down with the flush. Who needs incriminating DNA evidence swirling around in the master bathroom?)

The Poo That Betrays

Poop can be enlightening in other ways, too. Sometimes, though, poo tells you a bit more than you'd like to know.

For years, scientists argued about whether cannibalism occurred in the American Southwest. They'd found cut marks on human bones, but for some, that wasn't enough evidence. Then in 1993, University of North Carolina archaeologists unearthed an 850-year-old shit at a site called Cowboy Wash in Colorado. That poop contained traces of the protein myoglobin, which is only found in human heart muscle. Not only that, but it had been cooked first. (No recipes were found, to answer your next question.)

This not-so-savory discovery coincides with a period of severe drought, which anthropologists have blamed for the cannibalism. Other hair-curling theories involve warfare cannibalism, cross-cultural clashes, or even witchcraft. We'll never know which theory is right. We just hope the victor enjoyed the meal as much as Hannibal "I'm having an old friend for dinner" Lecter.

❦ DEEP SHIT!

Digging for poo may not be for you. Shit archaeologists tend not to have long careers. Unsurprisingly, the discipline isn't high on the academic totem pole. According to shit scientist Karl Reinhard, many shit researchers do just one or two coprolite studies, then move on to something a bit more "socially acceptable."

"What Have the Romans Ever Done for Us?"

Sad to say for New World residents, but long before early Coloradans were busily eating each other, the Roman empire had already established an incredibly advanced system of sewers and public toilets. As early as the tenth century BC, Rome had public baths and toilets, complete with sewers and flowing water. The baths were popular meeting places, and Romans weren't shy about lightening their load while chatting with a neighbor on a stone double-seater.

Some of the toilets even had a dozen or more seats next to each other. Not only was there no shame in communal pooping, but apparently Romans did not mind wiping with

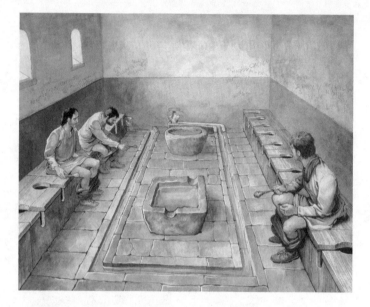

a shared implement. Titus and Lucius had the severe misfortune of having to share a sponge to wipe their asses; these sponges were kept in buckets of salty water for "sanitation" purposes.

How did the Romans create such an advanced system? They had the world's first plumbers. Highly sought after—as they are today—the well-regarded plumberi were often women.

Early Roman plumberi were so good at their work, their sewers lasted for centuries. In fact, one of the Roman sewer systems, the Cloaca Maxima, is still in use today, draining city runoff from downtown Rome into the Tiber River. In a foreshadowing of many subsequent years of organized crime, the early Italians even used the system to dispose of bodies—including, according to rumor, the emperor Elagabalus.

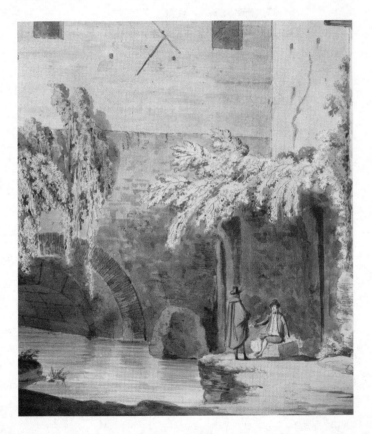

Great sanitation, impressive aqueducts, and shit leaving town faster than you can say "carpe faeces." What could possibly go wrong?

A Setback for Shit: Rome Spirals Down the Lavatorium

Managing a Roman sewer system took more than a few good plumberi. It also took an organized civil society, with plenty of workers and lots of denarii to pay the bill. Lose all that and what happens? The taps go off, the sewers clog, and you guessed it: The shit hits the fan.

And that's exactly what happened. With the collapse of the Roman empire, European cities fell apart. Even though cities like London had excellent Roman-built sewage systems, no one bothered to maintain them. So everyone left—in droves. They went back to the countryside. And when it came to shit management, thousand-year-old habits like chamber pots and shit trenches were back in a jiffy.

All that primitive pooping was okay— as long as everyone was spread out in the countryside. But after many years, cities once again started growing in size. And this time they were lacking all that Roman shit know-how. That spelled more than just trouble. It also spelled d-i-s-e-a-s-e and p-e-s-t-i-l-e-n-c-e.

The Dark Ages: When Shit Ruled

*"Dung and other filth had accumulated in diverse places
upon the banks of the river with . . . fumes and other
abominable stenches arising therefrom."*

—Peter Ackroyd, *Thames: The Biography*

With sewage systems crumbling, just how did you poop if
you had the misfortune to find yourself living in a crowded,
walled-in medieval city?

It was simple—way too simple, to be honest. Residents
would give fair warning by hollering "Gardyloo!" and then
would heave a chamber pot full of shit out the window. The
phrase comes from the French *Gardez à l'eau!* meaning "Look
out for the water!" This was a polite way of saying "I'm about
to dump a bucket of fresh shit out the window." We have to
imagine that it sent pedestrians hightailing it for cover.

KNOW SHIT!

"Gardyloo" eventually got abbreviated into *loo*, the British slang
word for toilet.

Medieval urbanites not lucky enough to own a chamber
pot or have a shit pit behind their houses had no choice but to

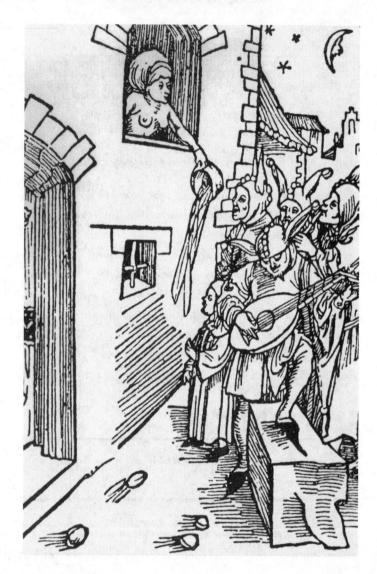

use a communal privy—very much at their own risk. It wasn't
unusual for someone to fall through the boards and meet a
particularly pungent end. Usually the poor mired serf was
lost to history. But not always. In one of the best-documented
moments of a major social faux pas, the floor in the Great
Hall of Germany's Erfurt Castle collapsed during a dinner
party in 1183. Emperor Frederick I and his knights fell thirty-
nine feet into a cesspit. Many drowned, but Frederick pulled
through—none the worse for the wear, though presumably it
was a while before his guests accepted another dinner invite.

With shit heaped high everywhere, you'd think those in
charge would build a few public toilets. But if you think it's
hard to find a public toilet these days, consider this: The
entire medieval city of London had only *three* public toilets—
Temple Bridge, Fleet Street, and Queenhithe, if you want
to really impress your friends.

Enough of This Shit, Already!

Shit in the streets. Shit in the gutter. Shit out back. Shit
flying through the air. After a while, even kings catch wind
of something ill in the air. In 1372 Edward III of England,
also known as the Disgusted King of Shit, had quite literally enough of all this shit. He issued a proclamation that
"throwing dung, refuse and other filth and harmful things
into the [Thames] shall no longer be allowed."

Ed was disgusted—and that in itself was noteworthy.

After thousands of years of not having particularly strong feelings about poop one way or another, we were finally making up our minds about how we felt about shit, and the operative word was . . . *disgust*.

So what? Well, as any poopologist will point out, it's the disgust that keeps us safely away from our poop. Which by itself is a good thing, given all the bacteria and viruses present in your average dung pile.

There was just one problem: just because Edward III was disgusted didn't mean there was anywhere to put the shit. More laws followed. But people kept shitting because, well . . . that's what we do.

In the end, though, Ed wasn't very successful at stemming the flow of shit. But he did accomplish one very important thing: His laws made taking care of your shit a matter of personal responsibility. It was no longer okay to holler "Gardyloo!" and dump a fresh bucket of shit on your neighbor. By the end of the fourteenth century, the fine for dumping the contents of your chamber pot onto the streets was two shillings, about $30 today.

What Shit Hath Wrought: Bring Out Your Dead!

All this shit was great news for rats. After all, no one loves a fresh steaming pile of shit like a rat. And European cities during the Dark Ages had plenty of steaming piles.

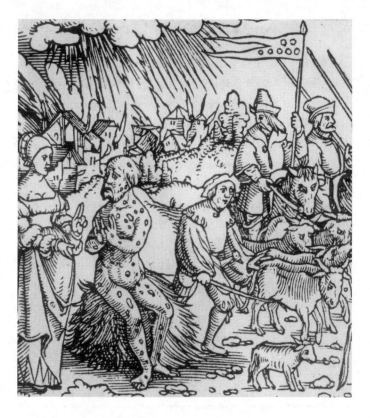

With rats came fleas, and with fleas came the Black Death, a series of plagues that killed as many as 200 million people—nearly half of the population of Europe. Then again, death might not have been such a bad option given the stench around the hearth.

Clearly something had to be done. Civilization was dying under the weight of its own crap. But what?

Plumbers to the Rescue

The unlikely heroes were plumbers! In the 1400s plumbers saved the day with a simple solution: the cesspool, an underground hole lined with brick or stone and porous material. Shit sank to the bottom and liquids flowed out between the spaces in the brick lining. Cesspools did the trick, keeping shit out of the gutter, in one place, and out of the reach of rats. Well, most of the time, anyway. There was the time celebrated diarist Samuel Pepys walked into his cellar only to discover that his neighbor's cesspit had overflowed into his cellar.

Of course there were still plenty of things that went wrong—like methane buildup, which led to periodic shit explosions, followed by fires. And cesspools smelled like, well, shit, thanks to hydrogen sulfide, and other gases, which could even cause asphyxiation, routinely killing people while they slept.

DEEP SHIT!

Want to re-create the stink of a cesspool? Just mix sulfur bath salts and hydrochloric acid from toilet cleaner. Voilà! H_2S, or hydrogen sulfide, the same stinky gas that killed thousands in centuries past. For that reason, we humbly suggest that you hire a professional and wear state-of-the-art hazmat protection if you want to try this at home! Don't say we didn't warn you.

Cesspools weren't maintenance free, however, and emptying them was grim work. Who got the job? It fell to the gong farmers—a phrase that literally meant shit farmer—an occupation that's clearly one of the least desirable in human history. As if gong farmers (also known as nightmen) didn't have it bad enough, they were required to work at night, according to this English regulation from 1562: "no Goungfermour shall carry any Ordure till after nine of the Clocke in the night."

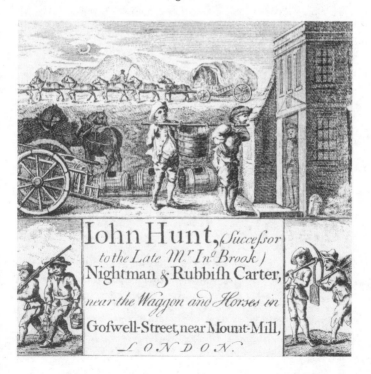

Once they had gathered their stinky haul, the shit farmers would dump the night soil outside the city limits in enormous shit dumps. The fee for this incredibly shitty task? One shilling, which few Londoners could afford. You guessed it: Cesspits hardly ever got emptied.

Deal With Your Shit, Okay?

Cesspools did detonate randomly from time to time, but at least there was a solution. Monarchs across Europe insisted that their citizens take responsibility for their shit. Edward III's dream had finally come true.

The rules were simple: Deal with your shit or face the consequences. In England, King Henry VIII appointed a commissioner of sewers who could mete out "severe penalties for the pollution of streams and made special provisions for the disposal of tanner and brewers wastes."

Meanwhile, across the Channel, conditions had gotten so bad that shit was heaped up in front of houses all over Paris. King François II issued an edict requiring homeowners to deal with their shit.

1539 Royal Edict of Villers-Cotterets
by François, King of France

The city of Paris [is in such a sorry state,] so filthy and gutted with mud, animal excrement . . . and other offals that one and all have seen fit to leave it heaped before their doors . . .

Sullied wastes and urines must be confined within the house and not tossed onto the street; they must be emptied into the stream and given chase with a bucket of water to hasten their course.

All persons are forbidden to leave any kind of unspeakable waste on the streets. Persons must collect droppings and wastes inside their homes, pack them into receptacles and wicker baskets, and then carry them outside the city and its surrounding area.

All proprietors of houses must install cesspools immediately.

A healthy dose of disgust, a rudimentary understanding that enormous heaps of dung just might have something to do with all those plagues, a simple solution—and humanity was on its way to cleaning its shit up. And it took only five hundred years!

Their Shit Doesn't Stink

Through these early years of shit management, one thing remained true: If you were royalty, your shit didn't stink.

As far back as ancient Rome, emperors had toilets crafted from gold and silver. At dinner parties, slaves would bring in silver pots for urinating; royalty would use the pots while at the dinner.

Later, Europe's palace rooms were appointed with stools holding chamber pots, called closestools or necessary chairs, which supported royal ass cheeks with a velvet-covered seat. These concealed chamber pots awaited the royal gift from kings and queens. The next time you find yourself sitting on the porcelain throne, imagine yourself scepter in hand, with your lieges before you. (Just don't bark orders to your imaginary servants so loudly you'll be heard outside.)

DEEP SHIT!

Grooms of the stool were employed by English kings and accompanied monarchs to the privy chamber in order to tidy up the royal tuchis. French kings employed porte-cotons who served the same function. (Could one overeager groom of the stool have gone overboard and planted lips on the royal ass, leading to an expression in common use today?)

Many kings even considered the closestool a throne and received audiences with butt cheeks firmly planted, thinking it was rude to leave a gathering to go to the toilet. King Louis XIV, who was known to entertain while his royal sphincter was engaged, went so far to announce his marriage to Madame de Maintenon whilst seated on his "throne," and English ambassador Lord Portland apparently felt it an honor to be received by the king while on the pot. Other English noblemen similarly found it an honor to serve the king while he was on the closestool.

What did royalty do when affairs took them out of their palaces and into their castles? The answer is garderobes, small rooms built into the exterior wall of a castle, complete with toilet seats that emptied right into the mouths of the hungry fish in the moat below. One hazard of using the garderobe—other than an enemy arrow into your colon— were the high winds, which sometimes blew the royal wiping hay back up the chute.

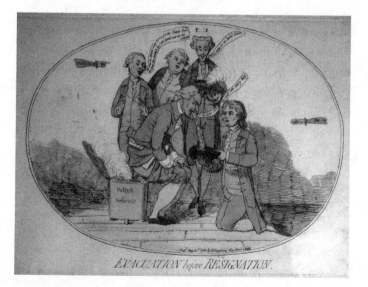

EVACUATION before RESIGNATION.

The closestool wasn't good enough for England's Queen Elizabeth I, though. She had a super-sensitive nose and in 1596 commissioned a solution, which became the first free-standing flushable toilet. Known as the necessary, it apparently wasn't, since its inventor, Sir John Harrington, only built one—for which he received a lifetime of ridicule.

All this royal fun and games came to an end with the start of the prudish Victorian era, when public displays of natural acts were frowned upon. Pooping was near the top of the list and was quickly hidden, ignored, scented, and generally denied.

The Big Stink

Imagine this moment in history. Thousands flee London. Those who remain lock their doors and hunker down, expecting the worst. Parliament debates closing its doors and relocating. Sounds like World War II, right? But long before Londoners had to worry about enemies in the skies, they faced an equally threatening foe attacking from below: shit. And until one wily Londoner saved the day, it looked like shit just might win.

The year was 1858, and London was in the middle of the Big Stink. The problem was simple: Sewage drained into the river Thames—but only during low tide. At high tide, London streets were actually thirty feet *below* the level of the Thames—a recipe for a world-class backup! To make matters even shittier, flush toilets were just coming into use. The massive volume of water was overloading London's old Roman sewers, and the hot weather caused bacteria to breed like never before.

KNOW SHIT! ❧

The stink was so bad in London in 1858 that Prime Minister Benjamin Disraeli called the city a "Stygian pool reeking with ineffable and unbearable horror." Government offices soaked their curtains in chloride of lime to manage the odor. At home, any aristocrat who did not escape to the countryside hung perfume-drenched sheets to mask the stench.

Fortunately, London had a secret weapon, the chief engineer of London's Metropolitan Board of Works, Joseph Bazalgette, who summarized the problem perhaps a little too clearly:

> At high water [the sewage] was pent up in the sewers, forming great elongated cesspools of stagnant sewage, and then when the tide went down and opened the outlets, that sewage was poured into the river at low water at a time when there was very little water in the river. [Furthermore, this sewage] kept oscillating up and down the river, while more filth was continually adding to it, until the Thames became absolutely pestilential.

Bazalgette got right to work on one of London's most ambitious engineering projects ever. Over a hundred miles of sewers were built over the next six years, draining all the shit away . . . to the Thames Estuary. This was no small project, requiring over 300 million bricks and moving more than 3 million cubic meters of earth, and on opening day, anyone who was anyone made sure to attend:

> *The Royal party landed at the Northern Outfall . . . and after a brief inspection of the works . . . the Engineer explained the general principles and engineering details . . . the four pumping engines were then successively set in motion by His Royal Highness the Prince of Wales, which completed the opening of the works.*

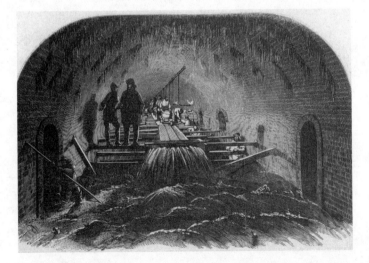

And as with every good British social event, "the company then partook of luncheon."

Fortunately the system worked. The city drained. And London had a modern sewage system—in fact, most of the system is still in use to this day.

⟡ DEEP SHIT!

The battle to tidy the Thames is being waged to this day. There are still sixty-three "outflow pipes" that still dump raw sewage into the river during heavy rainstorms. After rowing one day amid condoms, tampons and visible shit, one Anatole Beams founded the group RATS, Rowers Against Thames Sewage. Their first event? A Thames Turd Race, in which rowers towed giant shits while wearing gas masks.

Behind on Our Shit

When it comes to shit management, Europe's shit history was by far the best documented. Not a lot is known about poop's past elsewhere in the world. But this much is clear: Several civilizations beat Europe to the bowl, so to speak. And not by just a decade or two—sometimes by as much as a *thousand* years.

Take, for example, the city of Knossos on the Mediter-
ranean island of Crete, where a luxurious system was installed 3,500 years ago. Ancient Minoans had central
courtyards with baths filled and emptied by handcrafted
terra-cotta pipes. Flush toilets were adorned with wooden
seats, and featured the latest in overhead water reservoirs. It
was practically the first Club Med.

And the Winner Is...

The golden turd award in the race to develop a modern-day
shitting system, however, has to go to the ancient cities of
Harappa and Mohenjo-Daro, now part of India and Pakistan. Over three thousand years before Europe figured it
out, they were busy flushing toilets and had sophisticated
sewers, bathrooms built into houses, wooden seats—*even
coin-operated stalls!* (Okay, we're kidding about the stalls. But,
we have no doubt they're out there. Along with some shag
toilet seat covers.)

How did Harappa and Mohenjo-Daro get such a jump
start on poop management? Thanks to two things: knowledge of how to move lots of water for agriculture and a powerful government that could undertake big projects.

As it turned out, their two strengths apparently didn't
last, because both cities later vanished. Modern man had no
idea they existed until traces of their civilizations were discovered in the 1920s.

And that's the history of shit—almost. Because, lest you get high-minded about our contemporary Western shit management skills, your ass is in for yet another surprise. Consider this: Five hundred years before the western world even contemplated the idea of toilet paper, Ming Dynasty emperors had ordered over 700,000 sheets of TP in one year alone. The sheet of choice in those days was a gargantuan two feet by three feet—more than enough to make our old friend Mr. Whipple stain his trousers.

Shitting Through the Ages

400,000 BCE Mankind takes first dump.

12,300 BCE Oldest New World shit known to man left in cave.

2800 BCE Ancient Indus Valley cities of Harappa and Mohenjo-Daro debut flush toilets with sophisticated sewage system.

1000 BCE Not shitting is considered manly or even saintly. Indian scriptures explain that wrestlers who shit too much get weak. Saints, on the other hand, are believed to have no need to defecate because they can digest everything they eat.

(continued)

320 BCE   First shit management law passed: Athens bans dumping shit in streets.

600 AD   First use of the word *plumberi*, origin of the word plumber.

1281   Thirteen men take seven days to remove twenty tons of sludge from Newgate Prison's lavatory pit.

1500s   Revival of ancient use of shit as fertilizer.

1519   Government of Normandy makes toilets compulsory in each house.

1740s   Facilities for women are meager. Women are taught "virtues of control."

1832   Cholera and typhoid arrive in London from Asia, causing British authorities to engage in building public baths and washhouses.

HOW WE SHIT

There really shouldn't be too much shame in what you just did. You got up from the toilet and took one last look at your poop, didn't you? It was so close you could touch it. But you're not going to touch it. Thousands of years of instinct have taught you not to. We hope. If not, allow us to be the first to tell you, do not under any circumstances touch poop—unless of course you live in Asia; but that's explained in another chapter.

Certainly there are strong-willed people who don't look at their own bowel movements. But not you. (Would people who don't look at their poop be reading this book right now? We seriously doubt it.) Be happy that you are a normal person and, just like the rest of us, curious about your poop. We understand that there are times when you just have to look at what your colon has wrought, if only to answer questions like "Did I just rupture something?" "Did I just set some kind of record?" or "Did an internal organ just come out?"

KNOW SHIT! ❧

We each poop out no less than seventy-seven pounds of poo each year—about the average weight of a third grader.

For the previous thirty-six hours, you and the one-legged stool were inexorably bonded. Besides intestinal relief, maybe you're now feeling a bit of sadness for what you've left behind or maybe, if you treasure small victories, triumph.

But have you ever wondered how well any of us really know our shit. Probably not as much as we should. Let's address that, shall we?

Your First Poop

It's too bad we can't remember our first poop, because it was literally the last time our shit didn't stink. Your very first poop was meconium, a tarry, sticky substance that formed when you were just a fetus.

What's in meconium? Waste, of course—including a special kind of human fur, called lanugo, which grows on fetuses during their development. The lanugo is shed, ingested by the fetus along with the amniotic fluid, and eventually comes out with her first poop. Meconium is almost sterile and has little smell. However, meconium still looks gross as hell.

❧ DEEP SHIT!

In a university study, mothers preferred the smell of their own baby's poop over the stink of any other baby's poop—which is terrific, because the mother of a newborn is going to be seeing, smelling, and accidently touching a lot of her baby's poop. Less disgust may make it easier for mom and baby to bond. Researchers think it may also help mothers tell which baby is theirs.

If you don't remember your first dump, you might vaguely recall being terrified of graduating to the porcelain throne. You wouldn't have been alone—many kids experience stool toileting refusal, or STR to those in the know. It's not really a surprise, considering that you've just been introduced to a voracious whirlpool that makes everything disappear forever . . . and now you're supposed to sit on it.

As it turns out, most STR can be linked to pooping difficulties, such as constipation. Unfortunately for a kid with constipation problems, avoiding the toilet is only going to make the situation worse. STR can last for months, too—some kids have STR all the way to age five.

Which One of Freud's Personality Types Are You?

How is your refrigerator organized?

1. Alphabetically, then subdivided by expiration date.
2. Edible in front, substances altered by time and decay in back.

At tax time, do you . . .

1. Organize your receipts by category?
2. Start making receipts?

When giving a friend a present, do you . . .

1. Wrap the ideal gift in homemade wrapping paper and ribbon?
2. Drop a gift card in an envelope?

When you run out of toilet paper, do you . . .

1. Huh? Run out of toilet paper?
2. Improvise?

When was the last time you cleaned your bathroom?

1. Within the last twenty minutes.
2. If counting the rings in your toilet is accurate, it's been at least twenty months.

(continued)

If you answered 1 to most of the questions, you are anal retentive.

If you answered 2, God help you and all those around you.

Time for a Little Anal-ysis

Sigmund Freud, the Austrian neurologist and founder of psychoanalysis, observed that kids pass through a stage between the ages of one and two when their shit positively captivates them. The anal stage, according to Freud, is critical in determining your adult personality. It's all about whether you want to hold your shit in or push it out. Want to push it out? You're anal expulsive and tend to be messy, disorganized, reckless, careless, defiant . . . and possibly a bran muffin lover. Anal retentive? You're neat, precise, orderly, careful, stingy, withholding, obstinate, meticulous, passive-aggressive . . . and a more desirable houseguest.

In the anal stage, it is common for kids to play with their poop. If you're still playing with your poop as an adult, though, you're experiencing arrested development. Or maybe you just dropped your toothbrush in the toilet. (At least that's what you should say if anyone comes across you playing in the toilet. Also, let us remind you again, do *not* touch poop.)

❧ DEEP SHIT!

Here's something the folks at Pampers would probably rather you didn't know: Kids don't need diapers. Many kids in Asia are potty-trained from Day 1. How's it work? They wear pants with slits in the rear. Moms help their babies poop and pee by making the cueing sound *Hmmhmmm*, which means, "It's time to go," as they hold the kid over the toilet.

Hopefully, we've all made it past the anal stage just fine, though it's important to remember the words of Ernest Becker in his 1974 Pulitzer Prize—winning book *The Denial of Death*:

> With anal play the child is already becoming a philosopher of the human condition. But like all philosophers he is still bound by it, and his main task in life becomes the denial of what the anus represents: that in fact, he is nothing but *body where nature is concerned. Nature's values . . . are built upon excrement, impossible without it, always brought back to it.

Translation: It doesn't matter if you're an astronaut, a ballerina, or a zookeeper, you're still full of shit.

We couldn't have said it better ourselves, Ernie!

⚡ DEEP SHIT!

Prisoners, especially those in solitary confinement, have been known to play with their poop. Sometimes they're bored and it's all they have to keep them entertained, and sometimes it's a sign of psychological problems. They'll smear it on the walls or fling it at their guards. The official term is untidy behavior. Rumor has it, one infamous prisoner went so far as to make an entire chess set out of his own shit, which he played in front of others.

Now You're All Grown Up— And So Is Your Shit!

Each poop is different, its form affected by a variety of factors, like how much liquid you've ingested, how long your sphincter has stayed closed, how much stress you've been under, how much exercise you've had, and whether your sphincter is shaped like the star tip on a pastry bag.

Your poop has to start somewhere, and that's in your mouth. Not the most palatable thought, agreed, but it's all part of the process. As you chew your food and create a consistent mash, your salivary glands kick in and enzymes start to break down food molecules. Once you're finished chewing, your meal gets dumped down an organ that's all muscle—your esophagus, which carries that mass of chewed food, or bolus, down to your stomach using a wave of muscular contractions called peristalsis. Visualize how an earthworm moves, and you've got the idea.

❧ DEEP SHIT!

A lot of what we know about how digestion works first came from Dr. William Beaumont, who had a patient named Alexis St. Martin. In 1822, Beaumont treated St. Martin for a gunshot wound. St. Martin was left with a permanent opening in his stomach, through which Beaumont would drop food on a string and pull it out a few minutes later, to see what had happened. You think that St. Martin would have sought a second opinion after Dr. Beaumont left a hole in him, but then he didn't seem to mind being strung along, so to speak.

Think of your stomach as an enormous biological garbage disposal, where food is broken down for digestion and expulsion. Your mashed food is mixed with hydrochloric acid so powerful, it can dissolve metal—and in fact it has, at least if your name is Michael Lotito. The French performer, also known as Monsieur Mangetout, or Mr. Eats Everything, started eating a Cessna 150 airplane in 1978 and finished it two years later. His secret? An abnormally thick stomach lining and *lots* of mineral oil before his nightly snack.

To the Bowl—or the Body?

If your poop has a moment of conception, it's probably at this point, as your partially digested meal passes from your stomach and into your small intestine. It's showtime—when your body decides what goes to the bowl and what gets absorbed.

But how does food make the trip through your intestines? Again it's peristalsis, those waves of contractions of the smooth muscles that line your entire digestive system. When this action gets really powerful, it's responsible for that "10 . . . 9 . . . 8 . . ." feeling of the inevitable impending "delivery."

DEEP SHIT!

Need some action, and fast? Drink coffee! The caffeine in coffee is a powerful stimulant that induces peristalsis. Some alternative medicine practitioners go so far as to use coffee enemas to clean the colon. Unsurprisingly, this is *not* a benefit that Starbucks advertises. Imagine your next coffee emblazoned with this warning: *Please have a toilet nearby, as our product may cause you to rapidly deliver shit.*

Years of evolution have created a pretty smart sorting process, and it all takes place in about twenty feet of your small intestine. First, though, digestive enzymes come in from your pancreas and, along with the bacteria lining your gut, combine to finish breaking down the mushed-up food.

✎✎ DEEP SHIT!

Bacteria in your gut are killed off by antibiotics and chlorinated water, but they can be replenished with foods called probiotics. Examples of foods with beneficial bacteria include yogurt, cottage cheese, sauerkraut, soy sauce, and miso soup. When combined, these ingredients are known as the most horrible meal ever.

How did those thousand different kinds of bacteria in your gut get there? They were swallowed at birth—a little gift from your mom, you might say. It's a good thing you

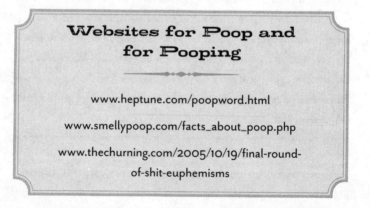

Websites for Poop and for Pooping

www.heptune.com/poopword.html

www.smellypoop.com/facts_about_poop.php

www.thechurning.com/2005/10/19/final-round-of-shit-euphemisms

have those bugs, too, because without them, you wouldn't be able to digest food made from plants. It's just another sneaky way your mother got you to eat your vegetables.

Once everything is digested, the sorting begins. Nutrients are absorbed through special cells, designed for maximum contact with passing food. What's left is waste and that's just been handed its walking papers.

Hello, World!

Before your poop makes its debut, it needs a few final touches, and those take place in your large intestine, a five-foot-long snakelike coil lined with muscles and mucus to help everything move along nicely. Here, just the right amount of water is removed to develop that classic, semi-solid consistency that we all know and . . . well, that we all know. At this point your proto-poop is still 75 percent water, 8 percent dead bacteria, and things the body can't absorb, such as cellulose and (as we all know) corn. Fiber is another thing that your body can't absorb, so that's why it's so good at helping keep everything moving along, like a little intestinal bulldozer.

The large intestine is where your poop-to-be spends the longest amount of time—sometimes as long as thirty-two hours! A wave of peristalsis contractions push your poop-to-be through your large intestine and onto its launchpad, your rectum.

Once it hits the rectum, the countdown begins. And sure, you can delay the countdown for a while, but poop waits for no man and soon enough it's time for it to "drop big," as the kids say. What a relief!

Ready, Set, Dump!

Ready to go? Great! What if you are, but you . . . can't? Sometimes it's not easy to find a place to poop, like at a new love interest's apartment or the coed bathroom at work. We've all been there. You *need* to hold it, it's just a matter of *can* you hold it.

❧❧❧ DEEP SHIT!

What causes that "I gotta go now!" sensation, anyway? Increasing pressure on your rectum sends signals to your brain to get the excretory process under way. You have a certain amount of voluntary control, but eventually your brain will hit the override button if it needs to make room.

When it's showtime, your brain tells internal and external anal sphincter muscles to relax. At the same time, it tells chest muscles, the diaphragm, the abdominal wall, and pelvic muscles to start contracting. If you're over a bowl, it's time to go. And if you're not? Well, you're about to experience one of those moments seared into your memory for the rest of your life. Please try to find a bush or mailbox behind which you can hide, because it can also be a psychologically scarring event not just for you, but for any eyewitnesses.

༺✦༻ DEEP SHIT!

When you gotta go, you gotta go! The late marathoner Grete Waitz endured two very public bouts of peristalsis while running in the London and New York marathons . . . and in front of millions who were watching at home, no less. Grete kept running, though, and it paid off—she won each race.

Let's See What We've Got!

And that's how it's done! You've just crafted a beautiful poop.

Now that the brown eagle has landed, you may want to take a look at it. Go ahead. No one is watching. (Actually, double-check that nobody is watching. You *really* don't want to see this on YouTube.)

In case you're wondering, it's okay to look at your poop. In fact, some cultures consider it a good idea so you can spot anything irregular. The Germans have actually gone

How's Your Poop Compare?

Average number of pieces: Usually one to three

Combined weight: Three to eight ounces

Combined length: Eighteen inches

Diameter: One to two inches

Shape: Cylindrical but tapered at the ends, like a banana

Odor: Ideally, should be only lightly odiferous. (A big stink may mean you're getting too much bacteria in your diet.)

Color: Shit brown

Float or sink: Most float

so far as to design their toilets with a poop shelf installed just above water level to allow for closer inspection. Of course, there are limits—when the psychiatrist in Augusten Burroughs's novel, *Running with Scissors,* encourages his family to look for signs from God in their poops every morning, he's probably taking things just a little too far.

In fact, the shape, smell, color, and consistency of your shit is so important to your health that shit scientists have actually created a special chart, called the Bristol stool chart, showing the different shapes of human poop, from painful-to-pass nuggets to explosive brown liquid. Check out your latest offering against the chart.

Bristol Stool Chart

Type 1		Separate hard lumps, like nuts (hard to pass)
Type 2		Sausage-shaped but lumpy
Type 3		Like a sausage but with cracks on its surface
Type 4		Like a sausage or snake, smooth and soft
Type 5		Soft blobs with clear-cut edges (passed easily)
Type 6		Fluffy pieces with ragged edges, a mushy stool
Type 7		Watery, no solid pieces. Entirely liquid

When it comes to color, our poop is brown thanks to the pigment bilirubin, which comes from the breakdown of our used red blood cells. The color of your poop is also influenced a lot by what you eat. Want to add a few highlights to your poop? Here are a few suggestions:

Green	Leafy green vegetables
Blue	Blue food coloring
Purple	Beets
Speckled red	Red peppers
Speckled yellow	Whole corn

You can turn your poop bright yellow by ingesting the protozoan giardia—but we don't recommend it, unless you're ready for a long-term bout of severe gastric distress.

Now, about that smell. On those occasions when you catch a whiff of something paint-peelingly awful, it's because your poop contains two foul-smelling compounds, indole and skatole. They're produced by the bacteria in our guts, and our noses are incredibly sensitive to them. Why is that? Scientists speculate that it might be that these compounds are also present in rotting meat—something evolution has taught us to avoid. In low concentrations, though, indole and skatole smell like jasmine and grapes!

Even if your meat isn't rotting, you still might want to go easy on the T-bone. Eating a lot of meat, which is rich in sulfides, may make your poop smell especially bad, giving vegetarians yet another reason to question the lifestyle choices of meat eaters. (Though, to be fair, vegetarians fart more—but more on that later.)

Poop Data

Average number of poops per day: 1 or 2

Average duration of a bowel movement: 5 to 6 minutes

Odd things ever ingested: A fork, $650 in coins, bedsprings, thirty magnets, tapeworms, a radio antenna, an engagement ring, sword, model airplane

Average time from mouth to bowl: 2 to 3 days

Fastest foods to pass through colon: Juice, soups, vegetables, fruits

Slowest foods to pass through colon: Meat and beans

Average constipation: 4 days

Top foods that cause constipation: Ice cream, cheese, beef, pork, pizza, potato chips, frozen dinners, hamburgers, breads, pasta

Top foods that cause diarrhea: Anything greasy or fatty, spicy foods, beans, corn, or raw fruits and vegetables

Percentage of Americans considered constipated at any given moment: Over 50 percent

Average number of bowel movements per day, men: 1.35

Average number of bowel movements per day, women: 1.17

Average number of bowel movements per day, vegan: 1.58

(continued)

Exercises shown to increase your number of bowel movements:
Jumping rope, brisk walking, yoga, deep lunges, squats,
bicycle crunches, a heated toilet seat

Onomatopoeic name for stomach noises: Borborygmi

Mission Accomplished!

They say that good-byes are never easy, but if it's brown, it's time to flush it down.

Maybe you pause for a moment and reflect on all that your poop has gone through in the last three days—namely you. Well, don't take too much time thinking about it, because deep inside you the process continues and no fewer than three poops are already taking shape right behind the one you've just pushed out.

With your poop happily excreted, it's time for us to turn our attention to a slightly more *explosive* topic: a little something that just might have slipped out in the process of making that poop.

KNOW SHIT! ✑

Kool-Aid used to feature a flavor called Purplesauraus Rex, which had a rather surprising side effect: It turned your poop extremely bright green. It turns out the dyes were reacting with bile in the intestine, resulting in a spect-poopular surprise. Sadly, Purplesauraus Rex is no longer on the market, having been replaced by a grape flavor with much less colorful pooping properties.

Poop Synonyms

A rumble in the jungle
Ass goblins
Ass kabobs
Baby
Black banana
Boom Boom
BM
"Brushing my teeth"
Captain's log
Chocolate channel chewie
Corn-eyed butt snake
Crack open a warm one
Dookie
Dropping the kids off at the pool
Droppings
Going dirty
Loaf
Caca
Crap
Doodoo
Doling the soft-serve
Duke
Duker

(continued)

Dung
Dropping a
  deuce
Excrement
Excreta
Faeces
Feces
Frightened turtle
Hell's candy
Hershey squirts
Keister cakes
Laying pipe
Launching a
  battleship
Lincoln log
Loaf
Load
Log
Making
Mank

Mank butt
Mississippi mud
  animals
Mud, Mud butt
Number two
One-legged stool
Parking the car
Pinching a loaf
Poo
Poop
Poopalala
Poopsicle
Potty animal
"Powder my
  nose"
Prairie doggin'
Scheisse
See a man about a
  horse
Sewer submarine

Sewer trout
Shitsicle
Splasher
Steamer
Taking a dump
Taking the Browns
  to the Super
  Bowl
Tangy butt
  nuggets
The fourth
  Teletubby
Toilet trout
Trots
The big job
Turd
Turtle Head

3

"IT WASN'T ME!"

You've almost certainly said it at one time or another: "It wasn't me!" But in fact it's even money it *was* you. As an anonymous eight-year-old philosopher once said, "Whoever smelt it, dealt it."

Let's face it: We all fart—prudish women, the president of the United States of America, sweet babies, your aging mother. Even *ants* fart. We've farted into our car seats, we've farted before peeing, we've farted during sex, and we've farted during yoga. Marilyn Monroe, perhaps the world's most famous frequent farter, passed gas during filming so often that directors had to work to cover up her anal acoustics. And like it or not, farting is one of the last things we'll do, too—many people pass gas after they've, well, passed.

Given that we each fart ten to twenty times a day, we humbly suggest that it's time we all learned the truth behind the much-maligned ass gas.

How, for example, can a perfectly routine activity have such a bad rap? It turns out it wasn't always this way. Hippocrates, the father of modern medicine, declared that "passing gas is necessary to well-being." For our fart phobia, we can blame those stodgy British. Starting in the eighteenth century, Brits began extolling the virtues of holding it in. Court etiquette pooh-poohed (as it were) the celebration of the body and condemned even the mention of bodily functions. Self-restraint became the standard among high society, while the common folk were left to pass gas as it so moved them.

Fart FAQs

Why do dog farts smell so bad?

In a word, sulfur. Dogs eat a protein-rich diet, and protein produces lots and lots of sulfur. Labrador retrievers, by the way, are the most fart-producing breed, in case you were wondering.

Why are dog farts often silent?

Have you ever seen a dog embarrassed by his or her fart? Neither have we. Because dogs don't care if they fart, their sphincters are usually quite relaxed . . . so the gas passes effortlessly. And noiselessly. And without warning.

KNOW SHIT!

The word *fart* comes from the Middle English word *farten*, meaning "to break wind." From the Latin word *flatus*, meaning "the act of blowing," we got flatulence.

To this day, flatulence is still mostly seen as a putrid, elevator-clearing nuisance. As undeniable as farts are, we're all still eagerly watching late-night infomercials for remedies, colognes, silencers, and underwear filters to mask, control, and defer our anal expulsions. The unspoken social proscriptions against letting one rip continue to be as oppressive as a fart in a spa's steam room.

KNOW SHIT!

In his forty-year career, Dr. Michael Levitt, gastroenterologist extraordinaire, has seen two patients who farted upward of 140 times a day. These overly flatulent folks turned out to be lactose intolerant. Once dairy products were removed from their diets, their gaseous anal emissions returned to the normal range of social acceptability. Says Levitt, probably the best-known doctor of farts, "Farts have been good to me. I've done very well, thank you."

Fabricating a Fart

You might think that a fart is born the moment your private toxic cloud leaves its anal incubator. In fact, though, your fart's conception started hours earlier, inside the inner recesses of your colon. The foods that are best for fart formation have lots of carbohydrates, such as bagels and pasta; our intestines just don't have the right enzymes to do a good job of breaking down and absorbing complex carbs. Foods packed with fructose are excellent, too, because instead of being absorbed entirely, the sugar ferments away inside your large intestine. Finally there's always that old gaseous standby, beans, which also ferment in our guts, giving off plenty of high-quality fart gas.

KNOW SHIT!

Burps are the stomach's version of farts, as the stomach releases gas that was created during the first stages of digestion. Fortunately for the purveyors of mouthwash and breath mints, the gas composition is totally different—and a lot easier to handle. We can all be glad we're not crinoids, marine animals whose asses are actually right next to their mouths.

If you don't have the right food at hand, you still have plenty of chances to let 'er rip. Exercise, smoking, and yoga can cause you to fart more frequently. If you like to spend your free time passing gas, try anything that causes you to swallow lots of air—chewing gum or chugging beer, for example. There's only one way out for all that air—and it's not through your ears.

Things That Make You Go *Pffffft!*

Foods that make you fart: Carbonated drinks, chewing gum, beans, broccoli, brussels sprouts, carrots, raisins, bananas, onions, dairy products, cabbage, cauliflower, grains, fiber, and pumpernickel—which means "goblin that breaks wind" in German

Activities that make you fart: Exercise, yoga, high-altitude climbing, smoking, chugging beer

Illnesses that make you fart: Lactose intolerance, colitis, celiac disease, Crohn's disease, diabetes, irritable bowel syndrome

Medicines that make you fart: Antibiotics, diabetes drugs, cholesterol-lowering medications, narcotics, calcium channel blockers

Hazardous Occupations

We've all seen our colleagues bend over at the copier and heard them let one rip. The sudden pressure on the intestines pushes out the leftover gas from Mexican night and forces your colleague to embark on the long walk of shame back to her cubicle. It's that same intestinal pressure in the yoga posture, pavanamuktasana (a wind-relieving pose, for the non-yogis), which releases the intestinal winds in a crowded room of relaxing yoginis. In fact, many yoga poses

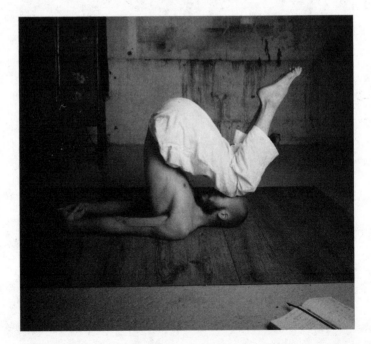

encourage deep breathing and the twisting of internal organs. Combine that with a relaxed frame of mind and body, and your butt will be roaring, "Namaste!" As the Ashtanga Yoga instructor David Swenson calmly noted after being hit face-on with a student's fart, "It's an occupational hazard." (And if you think that's bad, consider that in Bikram Yoga, incense is never used!)

KNOW SHIT!

Into enlightened tooting? Try the vajrasana, bakasana, svanasana, or pranayama yoga poses. Known as wind-relieving poses, they push out gas by stimulating the smooth muscles lining your colon and increasing blood flow.

DEEP SHIT!

Mountain climbers often experience high altitude flatus expulsion (HAFE), a gastrointestinal syndrome that increases toots at high altitudes. In one of the more unique medical studies of the century, trials atop nine-thousand-foot mountains in Bishop, California, confirm that HAFE is due to the differing atmospheric pressures between the inside of your body and the atmosphere outside. In other words, it's your body's way of adjusting!

When It's Time to Let Fly

Once the gas in your ass has reached critical mass, you're ready to let fly. Unlike the rest of the process, though—and much to the relief of Miss Manners—the act of farting is part of the voluntary nervous system. In other words, it *is* under your control. When you decide to release your per-

Fart Synonyms

Air bagel

Anal acoustics

Anal volcano

A turd whistling
  for the right
  of way

Blast the ass
  trumpet

Blow the big
  brown horn

Breaking wind

Butt trumpet

Butt tuba

Case of the
  vapors

Crack a rat

Cut the cheese

Doing the
  one-cheek sneak

Flatulence

Float an air biscuit

Fluffing

Gas attack

Invert a burp

Lay an egg

Let one rip

Low-flying
  ducks

Morning
  thunder

Pass gas

Rip one

Set off an SBD

The tree frogs are
  barking

Toot, tooting

Trouser cough

sonal toxic cloud is between you and your anal sphincter. At times, though, the urge to pass gas may become so great, that you simply have to let fly. As for those ones that "just slip out," fartologists aren't sure if it's simply a matter of training, or if our nervous systems aren't up to the task of detecting minor gaseous ass releases. However, one thing is known for sure: If you try to hold in farts for too long, you'll develop intestinal bloating. Try it routinely, and you actually run the risk of developing hemorrhoids!

🐾 DEEP SHIT!

For centuries, it was thought that holding in gas was bad for your health (and definitely bad for your breath). Romans actually thought you could be poisoned by your own fart if you didn't let fly. The Emperor Claudius took this matter so seriously that he passed a law legalizing farts during mealtime after learning of a man who had died, allegedly of being too modest about breaking wind at the table. His law stated that "all Roman citizens shall be allowed to pass gas whenever necessary." Then again, Claudius was infamous for passing up to twenty edicts a day. Incidentally, he was also murdered—possibly by a mob of angry Romans tired of all the smelly bubbling in the public baths.

Of course there are limits. You can keep a fart inside your colon only until the gas pressure overcomes your ability to keep your sphincter muscles tight in the face of great odds. If the involuntary waves of peristalsis contractions are too strong, your sphincter will lose out. Even if Kate Winslet is in the room and you were just starting to hit it off!

Fart FAQ\s

Paging Sigmund Freud! Why *are* farts so funny?

Freud thought jokes were very important because, like the unconscious, jokes strike a balance between what's expressed and what's suppressed. (And what walks that fine line in our bodies more than a fart?) We laugh when something sneaks past the censor in our brain that normally gets us to withhold certain thoughts. It takes a lot of work to constantly manage what's on your mind. When we don't have to do that, it feels great—and we release that extra energy as a laugh.

In fact, the world's very first joke ever, reputed to be from the Sumerians, about four thousand years ago, was a fart joke. Ready? Here it is: "Something which has never occurred since time immemorial: a young woman did not fart in her husband's lap."

Laughing your ass off? Us, neither. Humor's come a long way in the last forty centuries.

And what about that noise we all hear when the coast is clear and you can finally free your fart? The *pthh-h-hh-h* sound is actually caused by the moving gas causing your anal sphincter to vibrate. The quality of the sound also depends upon how strong your sphincter is, the speed of your fart, and the size of the gas bubbles. Big bubbles, created by gulping in too much air, make more noise than the smaller "silent but deadly" fart bubbles.

Deconstructing Your Fart

What's in that fart you just set free, anyway? You can think of any one of your farts as your own little snowflake, because no two farts are the same. The composition varies widely, but the main ingredients are nitrogen, hydrogen, carbon dioxide, oxygen, and methane. The nitrogen and oxygen weren't actually created in your colon; they arrive

Chart Your Fart!

Your Fart Contains

nitrogen: 20–90 percent; hydrogen: 0–50 percent; carbon dioxide: 10–30 percent; oxygen: 0–10 percent; methane: 0–10 percent.

from simply talking, chewing, and drinking. You might think of them as the fart's faux gases—just along for the ride. The carbon dioxide, hydrogen, and methane, on the other hand, are the real McCoy—they're created in your gut as a result of digestion.

KNOW SHIT!

If it seems to you that your farts are floating upward, you're right! You can thank the hydrogen gas in farts for causing farts to lift.

But all of those gases are odorless. So where does the stink come from? The remaining 1 percent of your fart is the waste from the microorganisms living in your gut, and it's that gas that gives our farts their room-clearing abilities. So you really do have an excuse. It's not *your* gas that stinks so bad; just blame it on the little guys in your gut. What's in that 1 percent? Plenty of extremely smelly sulfur, plus the compounds hydrogen sulfide, thiol, skatole, and indole.

All those gases can be useful when it comes to figuring out what's going wrong. Take, for example, one long-suffering farter who checked himself into a VA Hospital in 1998. This patient complained of flatulence so severe, he was farting up to 129 times a day, not only that, but his feces actually fizzed! To diagnose his problem, doctors had him

Fart FAQs

Does lighting a match really get rid of the smell of a fart? If so, why?

Sort of. It turns out that lighting a match produces sulfur dioxide, a gas that's extremely strong-smelling to human noses—in fact many times stronger-smelling than the hydrogen sulfide in a fart. So the fart stench isn't actually gone. It's still right there. It's just disguised.

Why do you sometimes fart when you pee or sneeze?

When you pee or sneeze, your sphincter muscle can sometimes suddenly relax. When that happens, the pressure inside your colon is greater than the power of your sphincter. The result becomes immediately clear to you and anyone else who may be in the room.

Do farts keep?

Unlike poops, farts don't stick around. But University of Massachusetts at Amherst biologist Lynn Margulis did discover termite fossil farts trapped in amber! When she and her colleagues drilled into the bubbles trapped in the amber, they discovered the bubbles to be filled with methane and carbon dioxide.

collect his farts in four-hour increments with the aid of a rectal tube attached to a plastic bag. To reduce the amount of swallowed air, doctors actually had him clench a pencil in his teeth for over thirteen hours! Researchers studied the composition of his ass gas to determine the causes of his excessive tooting. Their findings? From the abnormally high concentration of nitrogen, researchers concluded the poor guy's ass gas was a result of nothing more than too much swallowed air.

Ostracizing the Odor

Sadly, the lowly fart has seen more than its share of discrimination, as has the farter. Through the centuries, it's been concealed, suppressed, and squashed by virtually every society. And the owner of said emissions? He or she has been the, ahem, butt of jokes or the subject of silent disdain. Worst of all, he has sometimes been forced into blaming the dog.

The taboo against farting dates back over four hundred years. Europe was just coming out of a few centuries of plagues, shit-strewn streets, and general bad manners. The Renaissance was flourishing—and that meant that all bodily functions, from shit to sex, were strictly taboo. That included the fart, as one Edward de Vere, the seventeenth Earl of Oxford, found out. He cut the cheese while swearing loyalty to Queen Elizabeth I and was so embarrassed by the action that he retreated into *seven years* of self-imposed exile. The next time he saw the queen, she was reported to have reassured him: "My Lord, I had quite forgotten the fart."

Other cultures joined in the gaseous repression, including nineteenth-century Japan, where flatulence was seen as repulsive and unladylike—so much so that married women were not allowed to fart in public *or* in front of their husbands. And if they did? That was ample grounds for shipping your spouse back to Mom and Dad.

Have things improved for the farter? Definitely! But not everywhere. Take, for example, the region of Balochistan, in the border region of Afghanistan, Pakistan, and Iran. To this day, residents consider farting in public to be the worst of all sins. In fact, in the early 1990s, a Baloch boy from the town of Usta Muhammad committed suicide after farting in public during a volleyball match. Three years later (and no, we aren't making this up, either—unfortunately), the exact same public ignomy befell his brother, who also offed himself.

✤✤ DEEP SHIT!

The Baloch people actually have a bedtime fable about farting in public. It goes like this. Once a father farted and left his village in shame. Years later, he returned during darkest night to peer in the window of his house and see his children. He tiptoed up to the window and peered inside. What did he find? His wife cursing his name, remembering that gaseous moment of infamy. The end.

Foiling Farts

With farting frowned upon, it was only a matter of time before ingenious inventors turned their attention to taming the uncouth fart. Feeling a bit too farty? Try one of these fixes, but don't come to us when you have to explain that charcoal pad atop your office chair to your coworkers.

Beano: Beano is a tablet that contains a human digestive enzyme, alpha galactosidase, that helps break down complex carbs so they're easier to digest. But Beano digests only beans, fruits, and veggies, so it won't help any gas caused by dairy products.

Lactaid: For those of you with dairy-based ass gas, you'll need the enzyme lactase to help you break down that food that your stomach finds entirely indigestible. That's where Lactaid comes in—in fact, it's nothing more than a solid version of the enzyme lactase. Swallow it at the same time as that aged Gruyère, because your stomach will need it on hand before the anaerobic bacteria in the large intestine turns it into a fusillade of stinky world-class farts.

Flatulence Deodorizer Pads: These charcoal pads fit discreetly between your ass and your undies. Downside? The ten pieces of adhesive tape used to attach each one. And of course

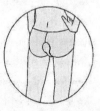

the box atop your dresser, labeled Flatulence Deodorizer Pads.

Charcoal Chair Pad: For those of you—and you know who you are—who silence the blast by squeezing your cheeks firmly into your chair, there's the activated charcoal pad. Downside: It eliminates only 60 percent of the odor, so that coworker with the acute sense of smell will still cast a glance your way, knowing full well who dealt it.

Fraudulent Facts About the Fart

As if it weren't enough for the lowly fart to be squashed, silenced, and aggressively repressed, our gaseous anal friend has also been thoroughly misunderstood. In the interest of honestly exploring our emissions, the authors are pleased to root out the truth behind the seven top fart myths.

Myth 1: Men fart more than women.

Status: True!

On average, men release more farts than women—ten times a day, compared to eight for women. But the overall volume of gas is just about equal. Women just tend to hold farts in longer, which means fewer releases, but longer, more potent and gaseous ones. A dubious trade-off—but it's your call, ladies!

KNOW SHIT! ❧

In an attempt to resolve many marital disputes over who lets it rip more, an Australian research team studied a group of men and women over several months. Volunteer sniffers were blindfolded and asked to rank the potency of farts, which were actually collected through a rectal tube and stored in aluminum bags. When researchers measured the sulfur concentration in the bags, the women won. But honestly, it was a pyrrhic victory. If you catch our drift.

Myth 2: A silent fart is a deadly fart.

Status: True!

Much of the noise from farts comes from the bursting of the fart gas bubbles. The bubbles can be large or small. Large fart bubbles are mostly air that you've swallowed, but the smaller ones are truly deadly, produced by the gas from bacterial fermentation inside your colon.

Myth 3: You can die from breathing farts.

Status: False!

As long as you're not breathing *only* fart gas! To get the 1,000 parts per million of hydrogen sulfide necessary to kill a person, you'd have to breathe *only* fart gas—and for six to eight minutes. Frankly, death would be an improvement.

Myth 4: Farts really are explosive.

Status: Sometimes true.

Only about a third of all farts are explosive. Those special farts need to contain methane, a gas that only some of us produce. How do you know if you're one of the lucky ones? You'll need to be tested for methanogens, a microorganism, which lives in the guts of five out of nine of us, according to one study. Methanogens are most common in ruminants (cows, for example) and are responsible for a large portion of biogenic methane in the atmosphere. So if you do have methanogens in your gut, you'll want to consider other ways to limit your greenhouse gas emissions. The chosen few who are able to create methane just need a match to start lighting up the popular "blue angels" and begin being the life of the party.

Myth 5: Your ass can explode from lighting a fart.

Status: Not *yet* true.

It's highly unlikely, but the flame could get sucked in and follow the methane back to its colonic source. The exact odds are unknown, the authors being unable to find any victims who told the truth to the attending emergency room physician.

Myth 6: Sometimes when you fart, a little bit of poop comes out.

Status: True!

Known colloquially as the brown pants fart or the Hershey squirt, the fart-poop hybrid leaves a bit of poop in your trousers. How does this forlorn moment come to pass? The nerve endings in your ass, which are usually quite good at distinguishing between fart and poop, can get confused when your poop is mostly liquid. The results? Take a look for yourself!

Warning: The fart-poop hybrid usually occurs when you're suffering from diarrhea or trying too hard to fart. If your fart has some poop solids in it, these are likely to become airborne and may stick to an electrically charged surface, such as clothing. Or your computer monitor. Something to consider, the next time you dust off your screen.

Myth 7: Your poop floats because it has fart gas in it.

Status: True!

Poop is heavier than water . . . most of the time. The fabled floater poop is the exception. It's buoyant for one reason, and one reason only: Fart gas is trapped inside.

Farts in the Arts

Though never fully appreciated through history, the fart has found friends among writers and painters. Here are the finest moments of farts in the arts. As to what prompted such moments of flatulent inspiration, we will never know for sure. But we're guessing it had something to do with that bean burrito for lunch.

Farting even plays a role in what many consider to be the greatest novel ever written—James Joyce's *Ulysses*. At the close of chapter 11, the character Leopold Bloom suddenly lets fly with an earth-shattering fart—concealed, luckily for him, by a passing tram.

✈ DEEP SHIT!

Farting was never far from Joyce's thoughts. He became infamous for his farting fetish, known as *eproctophilia*, expressed through erotic letters to his wife in 1909 about her flatulence during sex. No word about how the fart dispatches were received—but the Joyces were together for nearly forty years.

Farting's literary zenith, however, came early on—in Dante's *Divine Comedy*, written in the early fourteenth century. In the eighth circle of Hell, Dante and Virgil come across demons who fart. Or, who in Dante's words make "trumpets of their asses."

A century later, English author Geoffrey Chaucer gets a little more graphic. In *The Canterbury Tales*, the character Nicholas hangs his ass out a window and farts in the face of his rival—who then sears Nicholas's bum with a red-hot poker.

Our Founding Farter

Into this farting frenzy strode none other than the august Benjamin Franklin. In 1776, our flatulent founding father published a book of bawdy essays entitled—and no, we are not making this up—*Fart Proudly*. Rarely cited by Franklin scholars, *Fart Proudly* is a towering tome among the "freedom

Founding Farters

It is universally well known, that in digesting our common food, there is created or produced in the bowels of human creatures, a great quantity of wind . . . That the permitting this Air to escape and mix with the atmosphere, is usually offensive to the Company, from the fetid smell that accompanies it. That all well-bred People therefore, to avoid giving such offence, forcibly restrain the efforts of nature to discharge that wind. That so retained contrary to Nature, it not only gives frequently great present pain, but occasions future diseases such as habitual cholics, ruptures, tympanies, &c., often destructive of the constitution and sometimes of life itself.

—Benjamin Franklin's *Fart Proudly*

to fart" crowd. Franklin hit the sphincter on the hole when he stated, "Were it not for the odiously offensive smell accompanying such escapes, polite people would probably be under no more restraint in discharging such wind in company, than they are in spitting, or in blowing their noses."

KNOW SHIT!

The great masters weren't about to be left out of the fun, either. Hieronymus Bosch's *The Garden of Earthly Delights* shows a young woman with red roses shooting out of her derriere.

Thankfully for our young nation, Franklin wasn't farting when he was flying his electrically charged kite, or the results might have been catastrophic for Ben. And though he may have discovered electricity, figured out weather patterns, and helped craft our nation's Constitution, this founding farter never fulfilled one of his life's great ambitions:

My prize question therefore should be, to discover some drug wholesome and not disagreeable, to be mixed with our common food, or sauces, that shall render the natural discharges, of wind from our bodies, not only inoffensive, but agreeable as Perfumes.

Finally:
A Few Famous Farters

Though one of the most repressed of bodily functions, the Bronx cheer hasn't been without its share of fans—including a few fart aficionados with some rather unusual skills.

Take, for example, the Bedouins. Topping World War II's code-talking Navajos and the "clicking" Bushmen of South African, some Bedouins were capable of, well, sphincter-speak. That's right. According to British linguist Sir Richard Francis Burton, the Bedouins gave new meaning to the phrase "speaking out your ass." Bedouins created a language of arcane codes and warnings through a series of intricately nuanced farts. Implausible? Perhaps. But Burton also translated the *Kama Sutra* and spoke twenty-nine languages, so who are we to dispute his claim?

The Bedouins, sadly, never cashed in on their anal antics. But Joseph Pujol, aka Le Pétomane (French for fartiste) found no shortage of francs in his assly antics. In 1892, he debuted a fart show at Paris's fabled Moulin Rouge. The Fartiste played a flute, smoked a cigarette, blew out candles from two feet away, and even farted "La Marseillaise," the French national anthem. His farts had a financial upside, too: At his farting prime, Pujol was the highest paid artist in France! He opened his own theater, the Pompadour, where he starred for two decades.

The Fartiste didn't pull his act out of his ass. In fact he

came from a long line of professional farters. As far back as the first century, performers "possessed command of their bowels, that they can break wind at will so as to produce the effect of singing." That was according to philosopher and theologian Saint Augustine who, we're guessing, would rather be known for his philosophizing than for his observations of singing farters. Sorry, Gus.

KNOW SHIT!

Many countries had their own flatulent franchises as early as a thousand years ago. Medieval Ireland had professional farters called braigetori, and in the Kamakura period, during the eleventh and twelfth centuries, the Japanese had Oribe dancers who performed fart dances. How do we know this? Thanks to ancient scrolls that tell the story of a fart dancer who cunningly tricked a rival into trying to fart dance. The rival, it seems, shat his trousers instead. Score one for the Oribe!

Lest you think that the job of flatulist has gone the way of the circus barker and the cobbler, we're pleased to let you know that this line of work is very much alive and well. Paul Oldfield of Cheshire, England, known as Mr. Methane, discovered his ability to "breathe fore and aft" while seated in the yoga lotus position. Not one to settle for the occupational title of flatulist, Mr. Meth calls his trouser trumpeting Controlled Anal

Voicing. And to what heights can Controlled Anal Voicing take a set of cheeks? Consider this: He's performed such hits as "The Blue Danube," "In the Air Tonight," and "I Got You, Babe." He even has a Christmas album, featuring "Winter Wonderland" and of course "Auld Lang Syne."

KNOW SHIT! ❧

While Mr. Methane can fart for a healthy fifty-nine seconds, the world record appears to go to a Bernard Clemmens of London, who managed to let fly for a room-clearing two minutes, forty-two seconds. To let you in on a little secret, though, you won't pass out from the fumes—these farts are a result of sucking air up a pipe before release.

For those of us who aren't able to catch Mr. Methane's act, there's always Hollywood, which has expelled gas faster than the cowboys in Mel Brooks's *Blazing Saddles*—undoubtedly farting's greatest moment on the silver screen, during which a dozen cowboys create a campfire chorus the likes of which have never been heard since. The scene is so well known that it's even considered responsible for helping the movie get selected for the Library of Congress's prestigious National Film Archives.

How did Mel Brooks create a chorus of farts among twelve grown men? Hollywood has its own tricks for producing farts on demand. Often directors feed actors greasy foods before a shoot and get them to hold in the gas until the right moment. To deliver right on cue, though, actors actually have air pumped into their butts. (Fortunately for them, there's no list of actors who have had this procedure done.)

KNOW SHIT!

In *Blazing Saddles*, the governor serves up baked beans for the infamous campfire farting scene. Writer Mel Brooks took the character's name, Governor Le Petomane, from none other than Le Fartiste himself, Joseph Pujol, aka Le Pétomane.

The Future of Farts

While our friend the fart has been the victim of many a joke, it may just get the last laugh—and from an unlikely source: a group of single-celled microorganisms named Archaea. These little organisms fart, turning carbon dioxide into methane, according to scientists at Pennsylvania State University. How do scientists make Archaea toot? By giving them electric shocks. The methane Archaea produce can be stored and used to power fuel cells, which might just power your next car.

Farting could possibly save the world. Think about that, the next time you glance left and right and let 'er rip.

Fart FAQs

What happens when an astronaut farts in space?

In a spaceship, farts actually propel the astronaut forward. The stink doesn't have astronauts running for their extravehicular activity suits, however, because the air inside spacecrafts is filtered with activated charcoal.

How fast do farts come out of your ass?

About 7 miles per hour.

Do vegetarians fart more than omnivores?

Yes, they do! Gas is produced by undigested carbohydrates—of which there happen to be lots in cellulose, which is found in the cell walls of vegetables. Once that food hits the lower intestine, bacteria there go nuts. The result is gas—and lots of it. It's good news for the bacteria in your intestine, and bad news for the partner of a vegetarian.

KNOW SHIT!

President George W. Bush loved a good fart joke—so much so that W schemed to have presidential adviser Karl Rove sit in a chair with a remote-controlled fart machine. Rove, according to those present, was nonplussed.

⇥ 4 ⇤

WHEN SHIT GOES BAD

During the course of human internal events, there are sure to be a few excremental complications. Life is always full of little surprises (rain, wildflowers); it's just that when the unexpected or unwanted involves, well, *shit*, the surprise tends to be a bit more unwelcome. We should all take a moment to thank our lucky stools that poop, for the most part, ambles through the colon in an orderly fashion. Because when it doesn't, things tend to get horrendously messy.

And that's exactly where we're going in this chapter. We'll start with the merely psychologically scarring and progress to—yes—poop-induced fatalities. You might think we're ignoring the mundane and concentrating on the more nightmarish poop-related maladies. And you would be right.

A note of warning: If you're a person who needs only to hear the symptoms of a disease to realize that you are currently suffering from it, then you might want to move directly to chapter 5 before you suddenly find yourself in the ER after diagnosing yourself with Chagas' disease.

Better Living
Through Science

It must have been a wonderful day at Procter & Gamble when scientists discovered Olestra, a fat substitute that had no calories, no fat, and no cholesterol. The additive was originally developed during research into fat substitutes that would help premature babies gain weight. But the folks at P&G decided that Olestra would be wonderful in snack foods. After all, fat-free products are the new alchemy. Why try to make gold out of straw when you can make the absence of fat and calories taste like fat and calories?

The first product to hit the shelves was Lay's WOW brand potato chips in 1998. The front of the bag proclaimed that the product was "FAT FREE," but the smaller print on the back was the bigger news. "This product contains Olestra," it said. "Olestra may cause abdominal cramping and loose stools."

Yes, as it turns out, the indigestible Olestra in the now more unfortunately named WOW chips let itself out the back door, so to speak. This phenomenon was soon to be known around the globe, much to the chagrin of the marketers at P&G, as anal leakage.

Of course, this is America, where consumers have embraced everything from the ingestion of tapeworm pills to machines with vibrating belts to stomach balloons if they think it'll help them lose weight. It's a free country, and a fellow can play Russian roulette with his undergarments if he so desires. Besides, a little leakage isn't going to stop us from eating fat-free potato chips, right?

✦✧ DEEP SHIT!

In writing about Olestra, the Center for Science in the Public Interest put it best when they stated: "Snacking should be a pleasure undiluted with problems like dirty underwear."

And it didn't. Did P&G stop selling Olestra? Oh, stop it, you're making us laugh. The U.S. Food and Drug Administration decided that Olestra-laden products no longer needed to carry the "loose stool" warning. Did Procter & Gamble fix the "backdoor blowout" problem? Hardly. Instead, the FDA decided that enough people knew the problems Olestra caused, citing only a slight increase in anal leakage—likely to the surprise of the twenty thousand people who complained to the FDA.

In response, the fine folks at P&G issued a statement to

"provide additional confidence to the millions of people who are enjoying low and fat-free snacks made with Olean." Apparently, all that was causing anal leakage was a lack of confidence.

An Olestra endnote: It's recently been reformulated and is now used to make ecofriendly paints, marketed under the name Sefose. The sucrose esters in Sefose makes the paint slide around more easily. Sound familiar?

KNOW SHIT!

Want to try some Olestra? We dare you! You can still find it in Pringles Light Fat Free Potato Chips and Tostitos Light Restaurant Style Tortilla Chips.

We can't put all the blame on Procter & Gamble for anal leakage and befouled underwear around the country. There are actually plenty of non-lab-concocted foods that cause the same sneaky problem. Potential sources include a diet high in meat, fried fatty foods, spicy foods, dairy, and caffeine.

Artificial sweeteners like sorbitol, maltitol, xylitol, polyglycitol, and the medicines Lipitor and Xenical can also cause anal leakage—along with the medical condition known as an anorectal fistula. (No, you don't want to know.)

Oh, It's Supposed to Do That

Then, there's Orlistat, a drug designed to block the absorption of digested fats in the human body. But if you've eaten that fat, where is it going to go? Out the back—and very, very fast. The medical term for this side effect of Orlistat is called steatorrhea, meaning loose, oily stools. If you thought diarrhea came out fast, just think how fast oiled diarrhea moves!

KNOW SHIT! ❧

Orlistat is sold as an over-the-counter weight-loss aid called Alli, which one reputable study suggested can help you lose three to five pounds per year. The major side effect? "Gas with oily anal discharge." Go ahead. We double-dare you!

What Did You Just Put in Your Mouth?

Whether you know it or not, not everything you put in your mouth counts as food. One initial cause of poop problems is the ingestion of what docs call FOs, or foreign objects. Of course, if the object makes the whole ride, in the end, it's still poop to us.

Swallowing foreign objects is actually relatively common, especially among kids, who after all think that 90 percent of the earth is edible. (The other 10 percent is their fingers, which can at least be sucked.) Other groups notorious for ingesting nonfood items include seniors and mentally ill adults.

KNOW SHIT! ❧

On average it takes about four days for a passable FO to make its rectal appearance, though a third of swallowed coins are still taking their own sweet time two weeks later. After three weeks, doctors prefer to remove objects.

What's most commonly ingested? Coins and pen caps, which fortunately pass through the digestive system without complications 90 percent of the time. For the less fortunate 10 percent of the swallowers, endoscopy or surgery is in their immediate future.

Foreign Object Legionnaires

FO stories abound. Here are two classic tales in the storied history of humans, mouths, and things that definitely aren't food.

Party On, Chris

Eighteen-year-old Chris Foster, a student at England's
Bournemouth University, was having so much fun at a party
that he didn't want to go home. To ensure that he couldn't,
Mr. Foster employed the only logic available to his liquor-
soaked brain and swallowed his house key—a Yale two-
incher, no less. Mr. Foster had drunk what he termed "a
fair bit," which to anybody else is a way of saying "enough
alcohol to make swallowing a house key sound like a good
idea." Mr. Foster obviously has some very good pals because
they waited *until the next day* before taking him *on a bus* to the
emergency room. Of course we don't know the whole story.
One of *them* probably swallowed the car keys.

It Has a Ring to It

The diamond standard of the FO community is England's
Simon Hooper. In an effort to economize on his upcoming
marriage, Mr. Hooper decided to steal the wedding band.
Romance, it seems, has not died, though it may have gone
down the tubes.

Mr. Hooper visited a local jeweler and asked to see a ring.
While the jeweler's attention was elsewhere, Mr. Hooper
swallowed the ring. Then this criminal mastermind
claimed that he knew nothing about the missing ring. This
elaborate plan started to unravel when police located the
ring with a metal detector. Next, it was off to X-ray. The

keen mind of Mr. Hooper continued to impress when he told police that the ring shape in the X-ray was, in fact, a ring-shaped piece of foil he had eaten. Police had him stay at the station for three days, waiting until he made a "full bodily disclosure." Did the jeweler disclose the ring's anal history to the eventual purchaser? You can bet your ass not.

Go? No Go

Constipation, as we all know, is difficulty pooping, or when it gets really, really bad, the complete lack of pooping. What's the big holdup? Your body takes too much water out of the intestines, thus drying up your poo and leaving you up the proverbial shit creek.

Constipation, it turns out, has a pretty colorful history. A century ago, it was believed to cause autointoxication, or self-poisoning. Ads everywhere battled this new demon.

Then there's the case of Sir William Arbuthnot-Lane, a Scottish surgeon and one of the pioneers of using plates and screws to repair fractures. Unfortunately he also pioneered colectomies, or removing a patient's entire colon to resolve severe constipation—such a bad idea, it almost cost him his career. By 1913, Lane's opponents had him laughed out of the Royal Society of Medicine and had discredited his solution of major surgery for constipation. The fate of his patients is less well known, though; presumably, they

Fiber:
Your Colon's BFF

It might be a good time to highlight fiber, the action hero to the evil villain named constipation. Fiber works because it does not get absorbed by your body. There are two kinds. Soluble fiber (including oats, beans, carrots, apples, citrus fruits) breaks down into a gel-like substance that keeps your colon blissfully lubricated. Kind of like a secret agent, soluble fiber does its best work in the background, coming up behind constipation and giving it a karate chop to the neck. On the other hand, insoluble fiber (including whole grains, wheat and corn bran, nuts, seeds, some fruits and vegetables) is the muscle. It travels through your colon, scrubbing the walls free of everything in its way. In the world of colonic superheroes, insoluble fiber kicks open the front door, roundhouse-kicks constipation in the face, and helps shove poop out the back.

Poop advisory: Before you go eat a bushel of roughage, know that you have to work fiber into your diet gradually. Too much and it will create gas, bloating, and cramping. You don't want a piece of that action.

had the misfortune of spending the rest of their days with a bag strapped to their midriffs.

DEEP SHIT!

It's a little-known fact, but the nations of Britain and the United States battled each other after the Revolution, too. It was the late 1800s, and the nations were vying for the title of Most Constipated, blockage then being considered the price our asses had to pay for progress.

Finally, there's the case of early constipation crusader Dr. John Harvey Kellogg, who went on to invent cornflakes with his brother, William. In his book *Plain Talk for Young and Old*, Dr. Kellogg advocated eating fruit and fiber to combat constipation, which is not bad advice even today. Of course he also suggested kneading and "percussing" the bowels every day and told women that retained feces was one of the biggest causes of their bad breath. At least he invented cornflakes.

KNOW SHIT!

The world's record for constipation? Twenty-three shitless days. The once-bloated holder of the dubious honor is Chris Orton of Madrid, Spain.

Thousands of Doctors Prescribe
Kellogg's All-Bran for Constipation

IT is terrible—the toll that constipation takes in health and happiness. It thieves beauty. It wrecks vitality. It is the cause of much suffering and disease. And all the while it could be so easily relieved! Kellogg's ALL-BRAN is guaranteed to relieve constipation—safely, permanently.

Doctors recommend ALL-BRAN because it is 100% bran. They know that 100% bran means 100% results.

ALL-BRAN carries through the system moisture which its "bulk" absorbs. And it gently distends the intestines—cleansing, removing wastes.

Eat at least two tablespoonfuls of Kellogg's ALL-BRAN every day—in chronic cases with every meal. Serve ALL-BRAN with cold milk or cream—and add fruits if desired.

Sold by all Grocers

KELLOGG COMPANY
of GREAT BRITAIN, Ltd.
329, High Holborn
London, W. C. 1

Made by Kellogg in London, Canada

Ad 4

Most backups are usually easily cleared, though laxative companies would like you to think otherwise. They've conned Americans into spending $725 million on their wares each year. It's just one of the many dirty little secrets of the poop-industrial complex. Every now and then, though, a reason comes along that's legit. Like, for example, having a huge growth in your ass called—we are not making this up—megarectum. Megarectum is not to be confused with bloating of the colon, called megacolon, which can also cause constipation. You qualify for megacolon only if your colon is more than twelve inches in diameter. Sorry, we're not making that up, either. And yes, we know it's a disgusting thought.

KNOW SHIT!

When constipation gets really, really bad, your poop can harden in your colon into a mass as hard as a rock, called a fecaloma. If digital disimpaction doesn't do the trick, your doctor will have to operate.

What's Stopping Me Up?

Dehydration, lack of fiber, a sedentary lifestyle, pregnancy, changes in daily routine, pain medication, abuse of laxatives, diabetes, multiple sclerosis, anxiety, Parkinson's disease, low thyroid activity, an intestinal mass, colon cancer, antidepressants, an injured anal sphincter, lead poisoning, lactose intolerance, quitting smoking, psychosomatic constipation.

↜❦↝ DEEP SHIT!

Elvis Presley may have died with the remains of a peanut butter, banana, and bacon sandwich in his intestine along with a candy-dish-worth of pharmaceuticals, but he definitely did not die with sixty pounds of impacted fecal matter clogging his intestines, as some Internet backwaters have claimed. For that matter, neither did John Wayne, Anna Nicole Smith, or any other posthumous celebrity with larger-than-life appetites.

A River Runs Through It

Diarrhea, from the Greek *diarrhoia*, which translates as "a flowing through," is known by many horribly descriptive nicknames, including the runs, the trots, and the squirts. The British spell it diarrhoea, as if adding an extra vowel somehow made it more prestigious. However you choose to say it, diarrhea tends to be the most unpleasant of surprises. If the need to take a regular poop registers in our mind like the beeping of a microwave oven, the one associated with diarrhea is more like seven rocket-powered fire trucks flying down a hill, sirens wailing.

There are a plethora of causes for diarrhea. Here, then, in alphabetical order are the highlights: Addison's disease, alcoholism, antibiotics, astrovirus (surprisingly, not brought to Earth by astronauts), binge drinking, blastocystis, candidia, campylobacter (truly a camp to avoid), celiac disease,

Who got out of bed the wrong side?

COME ALONG PETER, you can't deceive your mother. Let me see your tongue. Tch! Tch! No wonder you're off colour. Off you go and have a drink of Andrews before your father comes down. Surely you know by now when you need Andrews without me having to remind you?

It is the same story in many a million homes. They all rely on Mum and, when they're mildly out of sorts, Mum relies on Andrews. Pleasant, fizzy, laxative Andrews does four good deeds. Cleanses and freshens the mouth. Soothes and settles the stomach. Tones up the liver. Keeps the system regular. Yet, happily, Andrews is not habit-forming.

Next time you need a little help, get it from Andrews.

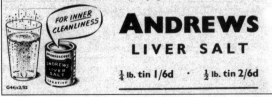

FOR INNER CLEANLINESS

ANDREWS
LIVER SALT

¼ lb. tin 1/6d · ½ lb. tin 2/6d

G44/c2/52

cholestasis, Cryptosporidium (perhaps the greatest unused acid jazz band name ever), cyclospora, *Escherichia coli, Giardia lamblia,* hyperthyroidism, inflammatory bowel disease, Isospora, lactose intolerance, laxative abuse, malaria, norovirus, pancreatic disease, pinworm, rotavirus, salmonella, shigella, short bowel syndrome, tapeworms, *Vibrio cholerae, Vibrio parahaemolyticus, Yersinia enterocolitica*—these last three quite possibly the result of a scientist's broken keyboard.

⚜ DEEP SHIT!

How can a doctor tell if your rectum is working? Unfortunately, they can't take your word for it. Instead, if needed, they can undertake a little defecography. As part of the exam, a patient drinks barium, the unholy offspring of a milkshake and a box of chalk. Then later in the day, the patient simply takes a poop while being X-rayed. That's right. Ever experience performance anxiety? Just wait until your doctor tries to X-ray you when you're pooping.

But Wait, There's More

As if constipation and diarrhea weren't insulting enough, nature has created an astounding array of ways your digestive system can backfire. Here are three of our least favorite.

Diverticulitis

Did you know that you can develop pouches along the inside of your colon? Guess what happens when food gets stuck in these pouches? (Are you eating anything right now? Stop.) Those pouches get inflamed, and the inflammation is called diverticulitis, a problem common in developed countries where people don't eat enough fiber. Diverticulitis can cause cramps, constipation, and pain on the side of your intestine. And that's just the beginning, because it can also lead to bleeding, infections, perforations, and intestinal blockage. You can even get abscesses in your colon. There are other complications, but we'll spare you.

Irritable Bowel Syndrome

Irritable bowel syndrome, or IBS, is the wild card of bowel disorders. It can cause diarrhea or constipation or both, kind of like spinning the wheel of intestinal discomfort. There are several reasons why you never want to hear your doctor intone the letters IBS in front of you: It's chronic, it's painful, there's no known cure, and it's a functional disease. That means there's actually no physical abnormality in the colon—the symptoms are a result of emotional stress. Women tend to be affected by IBS twice as often as men. Even worse is that the ultimate female cure for stress, chocolate, is thought to be one of the top three triggers of IBS.

Chagas' Disease

Here's one to stay away from: Chagas' disease. Fortunately, it exists mostly in South America. Chagas' disease is caused by a single-cell protozoan, and its effects include fever, fatigue, headaches, rash, loss of appetite, diarrhea, and vomiting. But wait, there's more. It can also cause swelling of the eyelids, enlargement of the liver and spleen, swollen glands, and inflammation or infection of the heart muscle. Nope, we haven't finished yet. What freaks us out the most is that the disease can get in and disrupt the nerves of the intestinal tract so that a person *stops being able to poop.* This breakdown of the digestive system can then cause the dreaded megacolon—and yes, fecalomas that need to be removed surgically. Feel free to shudder at this point.

Those are just a few examples of how your colon can backfire catastrophically, and they don't even count bugs that find their way into your food from—how do we put this delicately?—unsanitary conditions. (Indelicate translation: Eating someone else's shit.) There is good news, though, should you ever find yourself aboard the SS *Indigestion,* fighting the latest cruise-ship superbug. Lawsuits involving food contamination almost never make it to court because juries happily dole out large awards when the victim's attorney stands before them and says, "My client was served the shit of the defendant."

A FECAL TRANSPLANT
⚜ CASE STUDY

A few years ago, Marcia Munro, a Toronto resident who was suffering from a nasty superbug called *C. difficile,* received a fecal transplant from her sister, Wendy Sinukoff. Prior to treatment, Sinukoff collected her stools for five days in an ice cream container . . . which we hope was labeled *"Not Chocolate Ice Cream"!* Sinukoff knew that her samples weren't allowed to be frozen, so she took them with her in her carry-on luggage. Luckily she dodged additional screening, thus avoiding one of the more awkward conversations in the history of airport security. The good news: The procedure worked, likely saving her sister's life.

For You? Anything—
Even My Shit

As if megacolons, fecalomas, and IBS weren't enough, there's a poop-related disease that actually forces you to *eat* shit.

If the enzymes or gut flora that help you digest food die off, you're in for big problems, including bouts of diarrhea. The solution? You may need a fecal transplant to get your gut flora back. It's a procedure with a proud medical history, dating back more than two hundred years, when medical men were fond of prescribing shit—taken orally, slurped down, or even rubbed into the skin.

So who's the best donor for a modern-day fecal transplant? Someone with similar biology, such as a parent or sibling. That's right, if you think you've taken too much shit from your family, don't make a big deal of it. You never know when you might need a little more.

How's it work? Simple! A doctor takes a donor's poop, checks it for diseases, and then mixes it with saline to create a liquid shit slurry. You can take your shit through an enema or through your nose via a nasogastric tube. Reports say the treatment works quite well in fixing a patient's internal flora problem—thankfully, usually after just one treatment.

That's Some Good Shit

It should be pretty clear by this point that coming into contact with too much shit is generally a bad thing. Unfortunately, valuable rules sometimes go out the window during times of great desperation. Like, for example, when you've just smoked your last rock of crack cocaine. Out of money and ideas? It might be time to try jenkem, a drug made from fermenting your own shit, then huffing the gas.

While jenkem use has been spotted in Africa, it's not yet the next big thing here in the United States, where it remains the stuff of Internet legend. That's all fine by DEA agents, who don't know exactly how to prosecute someone willing to huff his own fermented feces. Said a spokesman for the Drug Enforcement Administration in Washington,

D.C., "You've pretty much hit the bottom of the barrel if you're experimenting with this."

KNOW SHIT!

Jenkem is known to shit-huffing aficionados as butt hash. It provides the user with both visual and auditory hallucinations—of what, we'd rather not imagine. Of course the hangover just might include diarrhea and gastrointestinal disease, so we hope the user found himself telling his buddies, "Wow. That's some gooood shit, man."

KNOW SHIT!

It's unhealthy to eat someone else's poop—but what about your own? Unfortunately, you're not inoculated against your own shit, since the bacteria that live in your gut can cause serious illness if they leave their confined home. Still want to try? (Some folks apparently do find it a turn-on, calling it scat sex.) Doctors would say you're suffering from coprophagia—and at a minimum, they'd also suggest you get vaccinations for hepatitis A, hepatitis B, flu, and pneumonia.

Don't Die on the Shitter

Admittedly, a lot of shit is out of your hands, so to speak. Megarectums and fecalomas may bring you to your knees. But there is one bit of wisdom that we can impart: Whatever you do, don't try too hard. Because in this case, trying too hard just might kill you.

KNOW SHIT!

Four out of ten sudden deaths in the home occur in the bathroom, where people die while attempting to poop—though you'll never read about it in the obits. This form of death is most common in the elderly.

On one hand, seeing that the average American spends nearly three years of his life in the bathroom, it should not be surprising that some people die there. How do they go to the great toilet in the sky? It's not the poop that kills them, but a strained connection of the vagus nerve that brings on a heart attack. As the nerve becomes stimulated it enervates the heart and the upper part of the bowels so the person feels the urge to purge. Too much strain on the vagus nerve and, sad to say, you're shit out of luck. On the upside, your friends will say that you went out with your boots on—without mentioning that your pants were around your ankles, we hope.

A Royal Flush

- King Edmund II of England, 1016: Soldiers of his enemy King Canute hid inside his lavatory box and stabbed him through the anus. This makes us wonder exactly where the assailants were positioned, or if they were in fact dressed as a pile of shit.

- King George II of Britain, 1760: Died on his water closet from a ruptured aneurysm.

- Evelyn Waugh, British high society satirist, 1966: Died of a heart attack while on the toilet. Ironically, Waugh was never a fan of toilet humor.

- Elvis, 1977: Found dead from a heart attack on the toilet in Graceland by his fiancée, Ginger Alden.

5

OH, THE PLACES WE'LL POO

For virtually all of human civilization, we've pooped pretty much in the open. We've pooped on the Serengeti, we've pooped on the Tibetan plateau, and we've pooped atop twelve-seaters, right alongside our fellow Romans. King James I of England even pooped atop his horse, not willing to interrupt his hunt. (We have to admire the king's sense of efficiency, but this has to be one of the worst indignities to befoul—sorry, befall—a horse. And yes, we're including pulling beer wagons and checking into glue factories.)

Unfortunately, shit's filthy. It carries diseases and other terrible things—like worms, parasites, and those little bits of corn from last night's dinner. But somewhere along the line we got confused and began blaming the shitter instead of the shit. No lesser literary luminary than Jonathan Swift pointed out this sad development when he lamented,

> *Thus finishing his grand survey,*
> *The swain disgusted slunk away,*
> *Repeating in his amorous fits,*
> *"Oh! Celia, Celia, Celia shits!"*

Who can we blame for condemning our own shit? It started with the Puritans, of course, who could always be counted on to find bodily functions disgusting. Their desire to hide said functions further reinforced the need for little rooms dedicated solely to pooping—eventually culminating in Japan's Sound Princess toilet, which produces artificial sounds to mask our now-embarrassing anal audio.

Thanks to the Puritans, we can't even talk about pooping. At least not like adults. Nobody ever mentions that they're "off to partake in a bowel movement." Instead, we relieve ourselves in "comfort stations." We "drop the kids off at the pool." Or we go to "see a man about a horse"—but thankfully for horses, not in the King James way. Some of us are so eager to bid adieu to our poo, we even flush the kids before we're finished hovering. (That's still the exception to the rule, by the way: Statistically speaking, *most* of us still look before we flush.)

This interest in blaming the pooper has created an industry unto itself that's focused entirely on creating private spaces for personal pooping. And conveniently, that leads us to our present topic: the places we poop.

⚡️ DEEP SHIT!

Speaking of looking before you flush, the Germans love to do it! In fact, it's considered a routine part of any smart German's daily health regime. They love looking so much, German toilets actually have a little shelf designed to hold your log until you bid it auf Wiedersehen. Germans adore their toilets—and hate traditional toilets, which, they claim, cause one to splash oneself. The downside? The water closet tends to stink more than rotting knockwurst and it takes multiple flushes to de-shit the shit shelf. And men, watch out! The German shelf causes serious splashback if you pee upright, leading some German toilet manufacturers to add stickers encouraging guys to pee sitting down. Headed to Germany any time soon? Here's what to holler when you're pooping in a public toilet: *"Mann, habe ich eine schöne Wurst abgelegt!"**

*"My, what a beautiful log I have made!"

A Room with a Poo

So who were the first humans to poop privately? Ironically, the one class of people whose shit didn't stink, at least not to anyone who wanted to keep their heads attached to their necks: kings and queens. The first recorded private poo

World's Largest Bathroom

Government officials in the Chinese city of Chongqing were fed up with no public places to poop. The result? A brand-spanking-new Egyptian-themed, 32,290-square-foot bathroom, with more than a thousand toilets. "We are spreading toilet culture," said Lu Xiaoqing, a government official apparently in charge of language translation mishap. "People can listen to gentle music and watch TV. After they use the bathroom they will be very, very happy."

took place in 1556. The secret shit in question belonged to one of the Mughal emperors of India. Tired of waking up every morning to relieve themselves in oppressive heat and dust, they built homes featuring luxurious bathrooms, or *gusalkhana*, replete with massage tables.

Not far behind were medieval monks, who performed their private duties protected by wainscoting installed between seats. Putting God's poopers next to each other turned out to be a great way to get rid of the monastic poo in one fell swoop. At Cleve Abbey in Somerset, England, for example, the local river was diverted to flow under an enormous room with twenty-seven toilets arranged on two floors. Medieval monks were given strict regulations on using the necessarium: "And he shall [have] the cells shown to him to which he is to repair when nature's way demand it, and he shall be told how to bear himself seemly there in sitting and departing, and how to satisfy the demands of nature with modesty."

✦✦✦ DEEP SHIT!

The English word *toilet* comes from the French *toile* or *toilette*, which was a cloth on which items for grooming were placed. That led to *cabane de toilette*, which was borrowed by the Brits to become "toilet." *Lavatory* comes from the Latin *lavatorium*, "a place to wash." As for who took the whole pooping matter behind closed doors? Leave that to the Scottish Presbyterians, who adopted the Latin word *privatus* meaning "private," and turned it into, *privy*. *Shitter*, meanwhile, comes from those of us interested in assuring absolute clarity in our communications.

While we're on the topic of word origins, we can't go without noting that word *shyster,* meaning "a con artist," comes from the German word *schëisser*, meaning "defecator." In English, we're just as direct, when we say, "You've got to be shitting me!"

Many of our pooping routines appear to have their first rumblings in the Middles Ages. Not so for the idea that the crescent moon was used to indicate women's outhouses and the sun indicated men's outhouses, however. In fact, that appears to be nothing more than rabid Internet speculation. Many solar-themed cutouts were actually present in early outhouses to provide ventilation, let in some light, provide some cheery decoration in an otherwise none-too-hospitable environment, and provide an easy way to open the door, in place of installing a doorknob. Besides, as one poopologist pointed out, in the rough-and-tumble days of the American West (or, even earlier, in harsh medieval times in Europe) would it really be likely that two identical toilets would be built side by side? As for the "historic" photos circulating online, many of them are only decades old, and century-old photos of outhouses show no crescent moon or sun symbols.

Bringing It All Home

Once again, kings and queens got first dibs on the next great advance in pooping, with a royal flush. John Harrington, a courtier for Queen Elizabeth I, gave new meaning to the word *throne*, with the creation of the first flush toilet. The year was 1596, and Harrington called his invention the Ajax, claiming that, "This device of mine . . . reviced with water as oft as occasion serves . . . will keep your privies as clean as your parlour and perhaps sweeter too."

Well, sort of. Her Highness's tush was impressed—but her nose? Not so much, due to one big problem: Harrington's toilet didn't actually keep water in the bowl. To be fair to the good Harrington, his toilet lacked an S bend, which would have kept the scent of fermenting poo from wafting around the royal chambers. It led to more than a few glances askance in the parlor. It would be two hundred years before anyone tried again.

❧ DEEP SHIT!

John Harrington actually wrote a book about his toilet, entitled *A New Discourse upon a Stale Subject: The Metamorphosis of Ajax*, in which he detailed the invention of his water closet and defended it against critics. A great title, certainly, but Harrington's real problem was that anybody with a sense of smell became a critic.

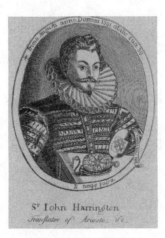

Sᴿ Iohn Harrington
Translator of Ariosto &c.

In one of humanity's notably slower timelines of progress, it took nearly two hundred years to figure out that water in the bowl and the now-omnipresent S-bend in the drainpipe would solve the nagging odor problem.

With all the pieces in place for in-the-house shitting, flies were suddenly no longer the only thing drawn to a healthy shit. Inventors, marketers, and scheming shit shysters rushed in to make a killing as fast as the new bowls could be sullied. Shit, it turned out, was gold.

The Poop Gold Rush

1851—George Jennings invents the first public bathrooms, as part of the Great Exhibition at the Crystal Palace in 1851.

1872—The French introduce the concept of the public pay toilet.

1880—Thomas Crapper & Co. Ltd. supplies Prince Edward with thirty cedarwood toilets and enclosures. The poop flushed very much like today's toilet, with stored water carrying away the princely "deposit." The addition of an S-bend pipe kept the stink to a minimum, too!

1885—Thomas Twyford, a potter, creates the UNITAS, the first one-piece china bowl.

It was a golden era for the porcelain throne. By the time it was all over, the twentieth century had arrived and bathrooms were in vogue from Newcastle to Neuchâtel. The flush toilet had a place of pride in the home. Pooping would never be the same.

Into the Pits

Of course it took many years for the benefits of the royal flush to travel throughout the world. As recently as a hundred years ago, farmers in the southern United States were still pooping away in their fields. The results were less than hygienic, with salmonella, cholera, and giardia running rampant. Poop diseases were so common that many scientists now think that the classic pokey, slow-moving southerner may have actually been anemic, courtesy of hookworms shared through poor poop practices. It was all figured out by one Dr. Charles Wardell Stiles in 1902. Working for the U.S. Public Health Service, Stiles wondered why southerners were so, well, *lazy,* and successfully made the connection with earlier findings that malaise-suffering Puerto Ricans were not sick with malaria, but hookworm. After years of trying to get his story out, Stiles finally crossed paths with the new Rockefeller Foundation, who liked what they heard. Doctors went south, asking questions like "Where do you poop?" (Answer: "In the fields.") "What kind of shoes do you wear?" (Answer:

"What are shoes?") "Is that a hookworm boring its way into your heel?" (Answser: "Reckon it might be.") The Rockefeller Foundation's solution was simple: Build outhouses—and lots of them!

✿ DEEP SHIT!

Rockefeller's outhouses were six feet deep, because hookworms can travel up to four feet. They were usually about a hundred feet away from the house and faced away for privacy. Some of them even had two holes—but not for company. One hole was much smaller to accommodate the little butts on the farm.

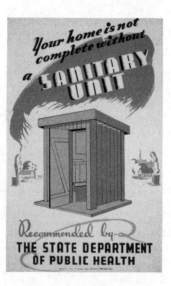

Your home is not complete without a SANITARY UNIT

Recommended by
THE STATE DEPARTMENT OF PUBLIC HEALTH

A decade or so later, Rockefeller's Foundation passed the shovel to Franklin Delano Roosevelt's Works Progress Administration, which went on an outhouse-building spree during the Great Depression. Teams of three workers would build outhouses for $17 each. And not only was FDR a fan of the pits, but so was his wife, which led to a nickname for the new buildings that couldn't have made her very elated: Eleanor's Outhouses. The WPA built 187,157 outhouses in total, taking an average of twenty hours per potty.

So . . . how'd they work? Like magic! They eliminated diseases left and right and left any remaining lethargic southerners plumb out of excuses for their slacking.

World's Most Opulent Bathroom

Pewter fixtures not chichi enough for you? Head to Hong Kong's 3-D Gold Store, where everything is—you guessed it—solid gold, from washbasins to TP holders. For a little sparkle, the owners have thoughtfully plastered the ceiling with over six thousand gems, including diamonds, rubies, and sapphires.

✵❦❧ DEEP SHIT!

Want to dig for buried treasure? Become an outhouse digger and shovel your way to riches! Outhouse diggers excavate old privies, looking for antique jars, jugs, and handmade bottles crafted from stoneware and glass. To get started, you'll need a spring steel stock probe three-eighths of an inch in diameter and five to six feet long with a T-shaped handle and a sturdy shovel. The best pits for digging should at least a hundred years old, before the bottling machine was invented—and old enough so you won't have any nasty, recent shitty surprises. Be careful though: Deeply buried poop that's not exposed to microbes has been shown to last for decades without decomposing.

Even if you don't find anything of much value, you will uncover quite an archaeological record as you dig your way through the poops of our ancestors. With the best poop, archaeologists can figure out what the poopers ate and drank and what ailments they had. (And when you do find that 1933 Saint-Gaudens Double Eagle gold coin, worth about $7 million? Don't forget the three coauthors who got you started!)

In case you're starting to feel a little embarrassed by our American penchant for pits, here's some good news: The United States wasn't the only country furiously digging pit privies. Japan, as recently as the middle of the last century, was a nation of pit toilets. There, pits were known by the four Ks: *kiken* ("dangerous!"), *kitani* ("dirty!"), *kurai* ("dark!"), and *kusai* ("stinky!"). All of which led a Japanese sage to coin the proverb *Kusaimono ni futa wo suru*: "Keep a lid on stinky things." To which we couldn't agree more.

Peristalsis Never Sleeps

Here's a reliably accurate observation about us humans: Unless you just polished off a pound of pure fondue, the chances are pretty good that before the day is out, you're going to want to drop trou and empty your colon. Which is all routine when you're safe in the office or at home, but what happens when you're rock climbing up Half Dome or El Capitan and the urge to purge strikes? Or what if you're busy repairing the Hubble Space Telescope and your post-coffee poop starts a-knock, knock, knockin' on your sphincter's door? Wherever we've gone, one way or another, some kind of toilet has gone with us. Let's take a look.

Profiles in Privies

LOCATION: *Airbus A380 Superjumbo jet.*

Toilet: Zodiac Aerospace Small Orbital Vacuum Toilet with Enviroclean Patented Chemical Injection System.

How It Works: Modern airplane toilets are designed to be as light as possible. When you flush, just a half gallon of blue sanitizing liquid is released compared to 1.6 gallons in a conventional toilet. Then powerful pumps actually suck the shit from the toilet, which is lined with a special nonstick surface.

What Happens When It Doesn't: Leaky lavs on older planes have been known to drop so-called blue ice from the heavens—which unfortunately isn't just ice. How does it happen? The unpaid load leaks, freezes to the outside of the plane, then releases when the plane descends to warmer temperatures. Unlucky victims have included:

- Peta Simey, who thought a bomb had gone off in her London home. Instead, it was a block of blue ice that crashed through her roof and landed in the master bedroom.

- Pittsburgh's Nina Cadmore, whose house got bombarded with purple, blue, black, and gray frozen clumps of aviation shit. No one would take responsibility—but a US Air crew did show up and scrub away the damage.

- A Spanish fellow who was minding his own business outside of Seville when a ten-pound ball of frozen shit fell on his car. The frigid shit bomb measured eight inches in diameter and crushed his car's roof.

Fun Fact: The first airplane toilets weren't toilets at all. World War II airmen literally opened a slot in their plane and let fly. U-2 and SR-71 spy pilots were even less lucky: They didn't get a potty at all. Wearing pressurized suits, they opted instead for preflight meals of steak and eggs, designed to bind them up until they were back on the ground. These days you still need to be careful about what you eat before your flight. If your poop is nasty enough, it may send fecal particles into the air, setting off the lav's fire detector. More than once a concerned pilot has ripped open the door, only to face horrendously foul air and a mortified passenger.

Disturbing Fact 1: Anxious smugglers will sometimes flush contraband down the aircraft loo on final approach. That's exactly why the Mob is rumored to run the aircraft waste disposal service at JFK International Airport outside New York City. Not infrequently they'll locate drugs, weapons, jewelry, and cash.

Disturbing Fact 2: A Continental Airlines transatlantic flight experienced "poor conditions" (their language, not ours) when a backed-up toilet spilled human excrement down the aisle *for seven hours.* The flight was diverted so aircraft plumbers could fix the problem; unfortunately, the flooding started again after takeoff.

The clogging culprit? A latex glove someone had flushed down the loo.

LOCATION: *Side of El Capitan cliff, Yosemite National Park.*

Toilet: Waste alleviation and gelling bag, aka the WAG BAG.

Use: Rock climbing, high altitude climbing, canyon-eering, and a really long road trip where you don't want to stop!

How It Works: Made of puncture-resistant plastic, the WAG BAG is actually two bags that come neatly pack-aged together. Need to lighten your load halfway up Yosemite National Park's 4,737-foot Half Dome rock climb? Just tear into a WAG BAG and place it over your ass—but only if you're confident that you have really good aim, because the WAG BAG doesn't come with a contingency plan for scraping your poop off the side of the bag. The inner bag contains a mix of chemicals to keep the stink down and also turn your poo into a solid gel for convenient leak-free transport. The outer bag has a secure zip system that makes sure your poo doesn't get punctured.

Why WAG your poo? Growing numbers of climbers have created a shitty situation in some places. Hikers at

World's Most Awkward Toilet

Probably the only public toilet to also be an art exhibit, this masterpiece is entitled *Don't Miss a Sec*. Designed by Italian-born artist Monica Bonvicini, the work "toys with the concepts of privacy and voyeurism." Made from one-way glass, users can see out, but passersby can't see in.

Guitar Lake near Mount Whitney can barely turn over a rock without finding an unwelcome gift from the last group. And on Alaska's Denali, one in three climbers get stricken with gastroenteritis because they accidentally ingested a bit of someone else's poo when melting contaminated snow or ice. WAG BAGs are now required at busy backcountry locations on Mount Whitney and in Mount Rainier National Park. Helpful rangers even hand them out.

What Happens When It Doesn't: Ever try to aim your poo? It's not so easy.

Fun Fact: WAG BAGs now have some competition from the Biffy Bag, a personal disposable toilet system. Biffy

Bag's big benefit? A burst strength of 50 PSI, to keep your shit from exploding inside your pack.

Disturbing Fact: WAG BAGs start to have issues as hours turn into days. After a day or two, the contents start to ferment, expanding the size and stink of the bag.

LOCATION: *Swiss train; Geneva, Switzerland.*

Toilet: AKW A + V Protec Bioreactor.

Use: Swiss SBB CFF FSS Intercity Trains.

How It Works: The current state-of-the-art rail pooping system is predictably a composting system in use by the storied Swiss rail system. Little do travelers between Zurich and Geneva know, but their poop will stay onboard for six months, making it all the way to humus, just a step or two from soil. The liquid waste, meanwhile, is treated with microorganisms, cleansed, heated, disinfected, and handcrafted into a Swiss café au lait that is simply *délicieux*. Okay—not quite. It's actually dumped safely on the tracks. We're sure the next generation will allow for direct source-to-beverage conversion, though. Any bets that the Swiss are already working on it? *Bien sûr!*

What Happens When It Doesn't: This is *Swiss* engineering we're talking about. When was the last time you saw a broken Swiss watch? We rest our case.

Fun Fact: Traditionally, train toilets simply flushed right out onto the tracks—a design called the Drop Chute Toilet. (Should you find yourself on an older train with a "Do not flush when train is in station" sign, well . . . you now know where your poo will be headed—right down the chute and onto the tracks.) As it turns out, pooping onto the tracks is bad for more than just the environment; it also wreaks havoc on the rail system. In fact the problem was so bad in India that scientists at the Indian Institute of Technology at Kanpur developed special alloy steel that resists waste-induced corrosion of their tracks.

Disturbing Fact: Old-style train toilets have a directional drain that's supposed to create a vacuum that will suck waste down. Only every now and then the pipe can spin around under the train and the vacuum can get reversed. The results? A fine spray of waste coats the inside of the bathroom. Nice, eh?

LOCATION: *Base camp, 17,590 feet, Mount Everest.*

Toilet: Luggable Loo.

Use: Mount Everest climbers.

How It Works: Invented by Nepali high altitude climber Dawa Steven Sherpa, the Luggable Loo looks just like a toilet seat on top of a five-gallon bucket. And that's pretty much what it is. But inside is a gas-impervious bag that makes it easy to haul poop off the mountain and down to warmer climes, where it will decompose, instead of staying frozen for decades.

What Happens When It Doesn't: The Luggable Loo works well as long as your hired porter is agreeable to hauling your poop for miles downhill. And it had better be downhill, too, because the gas-impermeable bag will explode if carried to higher altitude.

Fun Fact: After decades of dozens of expeditions per year, Mount Everest was turning into one enormous pile of poop. In the 2008 Eco Everest Expedition, Dawa cleaned up more than 2,000 pounds of junk—including 165 pounds of poo.

Disturbing Fact: Before the advent of the Luggable Loo, climbers at the Everest base camp would simply poop behind rocks. The area quickly became a high elevation desiccated poo minefield.

LOCATION: *Two miles higher, at Camp IV, South Col, 25,928 feet, Mount Everest—the highest elevation shit on the planet.*

Toilet: Open-air pooping on rocks next to your tent.

Use: Mount Everest climbers, waiting for the right weather for their summit climb.

How It Works: With temperatures of -20F. or colder, howling winds and altitude so high it's called the death zone, you need to poop very, very quickly to keep your tuchis warm. Climbers stay inside their tents until the last possible moment. As soon as they locate a stable flat rock, they open the specially designed flap on the rear of their one-piece GORE-TEX climbing suits so they can poop without exposing the rest of their bodies to the bitter cold temperatures and hurricane-force winds.

What Happens When It Doesn't: The entire process needs to take a minute or less, or climbers can experience severe debilitating ass frostbite. Blebs, or blisters, will form on the climber's ass—effectively finishing the climb for good.

Fun Fact: At Camp IV, nothing decomposes, because there are no bacteria alive at that elevation. Even Sir Edmund Hillary's poop is preserved forever at this camp!

Disturbing Fact: There's so much poop at Everest's South Col that climbers must travel far uphill and away from the camp to find uncontaminated ice to melt for drinking water. According to Everest climber Rick Wilcox, it's a routine fight among teammates to see who gets to undertake this unenviable task.

Pooping at Everest's South Col, while fraught with the challenges of functioning at extremely high altitude, is still easier than the climber's Camp III, on the mountain's Lhotse Face. There climbers have to use carabiners and webbing to clip themselves to two ice screws that are attached to the ice wall, then swing their asses over the 3,700-foot face . . . and poop. Your ass is literally on the line, as a fall would be unsurvivable. And the last thing on earth you'd experience? That's right—landing in your own shit. Well, yours and that of the other hundreds of people who have used these particular facilities.

LOCATION: *Presidential Inauguration, Washington, D.C.*

Toilet: Honey buckets and Porta-Pottys.

Use: Construction sites, movie sets, country fairs, all-day festivals—anywhere you need a toilet and one's not handy.

How It Works: Honey buckets used to be just that: five-gallon buckets that were originally used to collect honey and then got put to work collecting something much less sweet. Porta-Pottys are the modern fiberglass version, invented in Long Beach, California, during the 1940s so longshoremen wouldn't have to make the long walk to the docks with a heavy load on its way. The greatest number of Porta-Pottys ever assembled in one place? Five thousand in Washington, D.C., on January 20, 2009, for President Barack Obama's inauguration.

World's Safest Toilet

Worried about getting attacked by terrorists when your trousers are down around your ankles? This new public toilet in Beijing was designed after the terrorist attacks of September 11, 2001. Weighing over fifteen tons, the potty is fully bulletproof and even TNT-proof. The price tag? A mere $100,000—a bargain for those who want absolute peace of mind while releasing their own private chemical weapons stash.

What Happens When It Doesn't: Because they're so simple, Porta-Pottys hardly ever malfunction. However, the Porta-Potty is a prankster magnet.

Fun Fact: Before there were Porta-Pottys and honey buckets, there were shit-carrying street vendors, who used to roam the streets of the British Isles with a bucket and a large cloak. For a fee, the bucket would come down and the cloak would go up. We assume that for a few more halfpence, the vendor would whistle while your colon worked.

Disturbing Fact: Construction worker Travis Stone-house of Hazeldale, Oregon, was "dropping the kids off at the pool" when a tornado struck. Fortunately for Travis, he didn't end up in Kansas, but just a few yards away, unhurt—though apparently quite messy from the ordeal.

⚜ DEEP SHIT!

Have we inspired you to design the perfect toilet? Great! You'll want to test your toilet's flushing capacity, so to start, you'd better build the perfect poop. What to use for that faux feces? Poo researcher Bill Gauley tried mashed potatoes, mashed bananas, mashed you-name-it. But nothing floated or flushed like the real McCoy until Bill tried miso stuffed into a condom—and presto, artificial poo! How much to use? Well, your run-of-the-bowl poop weighs about 250 grams, or about half a pound. Most Americans, though, seem to prefer a toilet that can handle 1,000 grams—a true testament to the American love for supersizing!

By the way: the toilet test winner? Toto's Drake potty, which can pass a massive 900 grams of bean curd—a terrifying Godzilla of poo.

Even if you're not climbing Mount Everest, you still may be faced with a major poop challenge because the United States (like virtually everywhere else in the world) is woefully deprived of public potties. Fortunately, there's the

American Restroom Association (ARA), which advocates on behalf of the "restroom challenged"—those among us who find ourselves running for the restroom more desperately than our peers. As if that's not enough of a challenge, the ARA also fights for potty parity to eliminate long lines for women's toilets.

Still unsure if you want to join the ARA? How can you resist an organization that publishes a book called *Void Where Prohibited* and even keeps a tracker on their website showing how many people are currently tweeting while taking a dump?

The Final (Poo) Frontier

No matter where we go, our poop comes with us. And one way or another, we have to find a way to "have a debriefing" when nature calls, whether we're on the side of Mount Everest or stuck in 37C on an Airbus A330. Every toilet into which we've peered so far has had one thing in common: gravity.

Gravity, it turns out, is very important, especially when you want to distance yourself from your shit. Lose it, and you've got a dicey situation when it comes time to offloading your freight. It just won't stay in its container.

So how does one poo in space?

It's not so easy. Here's how it's done on the space shuttle, using the NASA WCS, or waste collection system:

1. First, float over to the commode and pull yourself onto the seat with the convenient handles. Don't forget to close the curtain so your fellow crew members don't have to watch you poop! There's not much room—the entire living quarters for a shuttle crew of seven is about half the size of a one-car garage.

2. Turn on the fan separator and vacuum unit. Then put your feet in the stirrups and fasten your body to the toilet with the pivoting bar—because what's worse than floating away mid-movement?

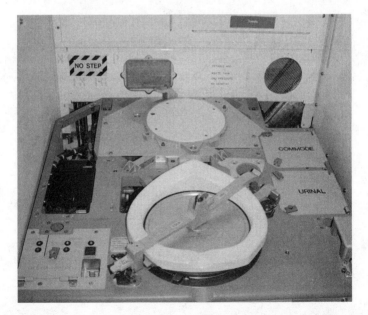

3. Carefully position yourself over the toilet opening, which is only about four inches by four inches. Why so small? The toilet actually sucks the poop away from the astronaut's butt. A tight seal is very important to a successful mission. (Good thing the training unit you used included a camera, to help make sure you're on target!)

5. Poop away! Remember toilet paper and wet wipes don't go in the WCS—the system would quickly fill up. Use the handy can.

6. Oh, and in the event your alignment wasn't everything it could have been, you just might—no kidding—have to manually push your poo with your hand. Luckily, gloves are provided if you'd rather not get that close to nature, if you catch our drift. As NASA shuttle commander Mark Kelly says, "You have to be really careful about going after what looks like an M&M in the shuttle. It might be something else!"

7. You're almost finished. Now it's time for the final check. Take a gander. Are you about to be followed out of the toilet? Your space poo should be floating down there with all the others. What's it look like in the toilet's inner sanctum? Says Commander Kelly, "It's not nice-looking down there. After a sixteen-

day mission with seven crew members, there's a bunch of turds there. They look like they're dancing with each other. Because they're in a vacuum and it's pretty cold, they're kind of freeze-dried looking."

What happens to the waste? The solids are compacted during longer missions, then returned to earth, where NASA auctions them at Sotheby's to raise money for the space program. Okay, not really. Of course it's all properly disposed of here on terra firma.

✎✎ DEEP SHIT!

Think being an astronaut is cool? Of course it is! Imagine sitting atop the shuttle as the launch sequence counts down toward zero. It's one of the most dramatic moments mankind has ever created. But consider this. Astronauts are in their orange pressure suit for as many as five hours. And, well, they need to be ready for any eventuality. So what are they wearing underneath all that NASA gear? Plain old Depend adult diapers, the very same ones worn by your grandmother. Sad but true.

Think pooping in space sounds hard? It used to be even more challenging—just ask the old-timers. Back in 1977, the Apollo space modules had no bathroom whatsoever. Astronauts used Apollo fecal bags, which looked remarkably like plastic bags taped to their butts. "You just float around for a while doing things with a bag on your butt," according to Apollo 9 lunar module pilot Rusty Schweickart. Cleanup wasn't easy, either: After pooping came the task of dislodging your poop without having it sneak away. All told, the process took about about an hour—about the same amount of time it takes Uncle Irving to complete the task after Friday dinner, coincidentally. (Though Irv's equipment is much less exotic.)

Houston, We Have a Problem

Of course when you're living on the cutting edge of poop technology, shit can happen. Like, for example, in 2008, when the liquid separator on the toilet for the International Space Station started to malfunction and nearly compromised the entire mission!

The Russian-built toilet was repaired with a new pump and control panel. The waste and hygiene compartment was operational again, and astronaut Robert Thirsk was able to proudly announce, "The WHC is go for nominal ops." What was the tab for that plumber's visit? We can only imagine it was out of this world.

From the final frontier to final approach, one comforting thought emerges: No matter where we go, plumbers have been there first. And they've thought it all through for us, from the moment when peristalsis perks up our assly nerve endings to the final wipe 'n' flush. And such progress! No longer do we trudge through the back forty to a chilly two-holer. Our cheeks are now caressed in decadent opulence, in rooms that have taken their place in our homes with pride. And that's a good thing, too—because just about three years of our lives will be spent in that room. Sitting. Thinking. Reading. And pooping.

❧ 6 ❧

AND THEN WHAT HAPPENS?

Okay, you've flushed the toilet and that poop of yours is gone forever.

Well, not really.

That poop whirlpooling into oblivion might seem like magic, but it's more like a magician stepping into a magic box. Ta-dah! While the poop might have disappeared, it's definitely not gone. (We hope we haven't ruined the magic box trick for you.) In truth, that poop of yours is at the beginning of another journey—an odyssey, really.

So now that you've gone, let's take a look at where it's going after you've moved on. First, though, let's take a side trip to consider poop's forgotten partner in the swirlage: toilet paper.

Pass Me That Goose: A Brief History of TP

Many a poop is accompanied on its downward spiral by toilet paper, its companion in swirlage. But it wasn't always that way. How did we get to that roll spinning effortlessly on its cardboard tube? Let's find out!

It all started back in AD 589 when Yan Zhitui, a Chinese scholar, calligrapher, painter, musician, and government official (who would have been a real Renaissance man if he hadn't been born before the Renaissance) was reportedly the first person ever to mention toilet paper, as well as the first to create the test for what could be considered TP. Yan wrote, "Paper on which there are quotations or commentaries from Five Classics or the names of sages, I dare not use for toilet purposes."

Wise words to live by and not wipe by.

KNOW SHIT!

François Rabelais, a French satirist in the sixteenth century, suggested that the well-downed neck of a goose was perfect for post-poop rearward ablutions. We assume Monsieur Rabelais never found himself in a pants-down situation while within neck's length of a befouled goose or her enraged gander.

It would be more than eight hundred years, though, before someone thought to actually make TP rather than fret about whether to use august literature to clean up. Again, China gets all the credit in the TP department—the records of the Imperial Bureau of Supplies show that in 1393, 15,000 sheets of special soft-fabric perfumed toilet paper was made for the emperor and his family.

To be clear, people were wiping long before TP arrived on the scene. So what were they using prior to the emperor's extravagance? Maybe the question should be: What weren't they using? Because it seems that besides your run-of-the-mill leaves and grasses, people were also partial to corncobs, rocks, moss, snow, water, sand, ferns, and, which must have been as painful as it sounds, sticks and seashells. It seemed that the sole criterion for objects to be classified as toiletries was propinquity—being within arm's length.

But long after Yan's sage advice, Americans were looking forward to the Sears, Roebuck catalog for more than one reason. In fact, up until the twenty-first century, Americans were still using newspapers, catalogs, and books to clean up their act.

Heady Days for Head Paper

Most auspiciously, humanity reached a time that we would like to refer to as the Golden Century of Toilet Paper Development, lasting from 1857 until 1942. Sure, that's only eighty-five years, but trust us, Golden Century sounds better.

It all began in 1857, when New York's Joseph Gayetty introduced the first commercially produced TP. For fifty cents, or a little more than ten bucks in today's money, you received five hundred flat sheets medicated with aloe and imprinted with the Gayetty's Medicated Paper name. While this paper was originally intended to help with hemorrhoids, it seems that people followed this chain of thought: "Hey, Gayetty's Medicated Paper, as long as you're down there taking care of my swollen veins . . ."

Not long afterward, in 1871, Seth Wheeler from Albany, New York, patented his idea for rolled and perforated toilet paper. And while it's not in the history books, this was also the moment that cats first took notice of toilet paper. In 1877, Wheeler's company Albany Perforated Wrapping Paper began selling and marketing standard perforated toilet paper on a roll.

KNOW SHIT!

Early toilet paper manufacturing left a little something to be desired—namely, there were still unprocessed splinters of wood in the TP, which must have led to occasional bloodcurdling yelps from the outhouse.

In 1935, ass-wiping became a much more comfortable undertaking, with the introduction of Northern Tissue's splinter-free toilet paper. Since James Chadwick won the Nobel Prize for Physics that year, we can only assume that splinterless toilet paper must have been a close second.

In 1942, not long after the introduction of pain-free TP, St. Andrew's Paper Mill in Walthamstow, U.K., invented

the first two-ply soft loo roll. It's good to know that shit research carried on even in the midst of a hail of German
bombs.

The End of the Roll

Sadly, there haven't been any great leaps in toilet paper development since 1942. It's still square sheets of paper that
come perforated on a roll.

However, that doesn't mean there hasn't been an assload
of innovation. Toilet paper manufacturers have tried pastel
tints, layers (up to four ply for the most sensitive individu-
als), quilting, and even medicated toilet paper, with a tip of
the hat to our old friend Joe G.

KNOW SHIT!

Colorful TP not "out there" enough for you? Try some novelty
toilet papers. Want to do a crossword puzzle? Sudoku? Interested in factoids about France? Well, there are toilet papers for
that, too. There's even camouflage toilet paper for people who
live in mortal fear of being spotted pooping by the neighborhood
deer.

One British company, Renova, even specializes in brilliantly colored toilet papers. And when we say brilliantly

colored, we mean shades of red and orange and lime green that could be spotted from the International Space Station. Renova's toilet paper is for those whose eye for design is daily assaulted by the blight of white TP in their bathrooms. And as an added bonus, the Renova website promises that the product is "colorfast for its intended use," so you won't have to worry about looking like the ass end of an African blue butt monkey when you're through cleaning things up.

In perhaps one of the more depressing bits of information for goats and sweater enthusiasts, Waitrose, a British company, has started to produce toilet paper with bits of cashmere in it.

Yes, But What Does It Do?

Maybe the biggest development that toilet paper has aided in the last hundred years is the concept of advertising a product without actually mentioning what the product does. Rivaling the code of silence regarding feminine products, advertisers have built an entire industry while speaking only covertly about what toilet paper is for. Perhaps no one is more famous in this regard than the lovable Mr. Whipple, the most famous toilet paper salesman in history.

Mr. George Whipple was portrayed by actor Dick Wilson. Starting in 1964 and continuing all the way to 1985, television commercials starred Mr. Whipple patrolling the aisles of his supermarket on the lookout for women (for the most part) whose inexplicable desire was to grope Charmin TP. "Please don't squeeze the Charmin!" he'd plead. Then having snatched said crushed paper products from the arms of TP-smitten ladies, Mr. Whipple would take a private moment to indulge in the same forbidden desire.

KNOW SHIT!

While Charmin commercials might not have told viewers the explicit purpose of TP, there might have been a tiny clue in the location where the first commercial was filmed: Flushing, New York.

After Mr. Whipple's retirement from the toilet paper beat, he was replaced with a family of cartoon bears. Meanwhile, Cottonelle's packaging sports an adorable golden puppy and Angel Soft has a baby.

What do bears, puppies, and babies have in common? They're cute. They're cuddly. And they all blissfully exist in a beautiful world utterly devoid of poop.

Are We That Full of Shit?

Thanks to Mr. Whipple and friends, toilet paper companies have done a stunning job at selling toilet paper to

North Americans. In fact, the United States and Canada are the largest toilet paper consumers in the world—by far.

Let's take a look at the consumption:

In Africa, the per capita consumption of toilet paper is just a tad over 0.75 of a pound.

In Asia, it's nearly 4 pounds.

In Latin America, it's 9.25 pounds.

In Western Europe, it's 30 pounds.

North America's annual consumption of toilet paper is 50 pounds per capita.

That's right, your average American or Canadian goes through 50 pounds of toilet paper a year. That's a whopping 7.25 billion rolls of toilet paper.

Big deal, right? Well, it turns out, even before it gets used, TP has a dark side.

Just One More Roll, Then I'll Quit, I Swear

When it comes down to America's burgeoning use of toilet paper, we can condemn the influence of puppies and cartoon bears—go ahead, it's fun—but in the end, any blame comes down on our metaphorical heads and literal butts. Why? Americans have become addicted to softness. (Don't think we've forgotten you, Canada. It's your fault, too.)

What's the problem with triple quilting? As Dr. Allen

Hershkowitz of the Natural Resources Defense Council says, "Softness equals ecological destruction." In short, we're literally wiping out the trees.

DEEP SHIT!

Musician Sheryl Crow famously suggested using only one square per restroom visit, except of course on those pesky occasions where two to three could be required. This created some furor from people who felt that Crow was claiming not only that her shit doesn't stink, but also that it apparently doesn't stick. Crow later claimed that she was joking. But whether she was kidding or whether she is in fact a one-square dabber, she did bring up one possible solution to America's TP addiction. Would Crow's suggestion have gone over any better if she had thought a little more outside the roll, and suggested tidying up Asian style with a squirt of water, instead? We'll never know.

You see, to create the downiest toilet paper, paper companies need to use a mix of long fibers from softwoods like pine and spruce, which they can lay out and fluff, as well as shorter fibers from hardwoods like maple and oak. According to Dr. Al, more than 98 percent of the 7.25 billion toilet paper rolls sold in America come from virgin wood. And, to get there, Americans have to cut down a tree for every 2 poopers, or about 150 million trees a year. And that's not counting Canada. (See, Canadians, we didn't forget you.)

Now, as poopologists we should remain nonpartisan on the subject, but holy crap, that seems like a lot, doesn't it?

Reduce, Reuse, Recycle?

We can't reduce our quantity of poop—at least not without drastic measures, like massively increasing our cheese intake. And we can't reuse toilet paper. (Have you tried? It's not so easy.) However, we can recycle. Sort of. According to the Natural Resources Defense Council, if every household in the United States replaced one 500-sheet roll of virgin fiber toilet paper ("But it's so soft!" Yes, yes, we know) with a 100 percent recycled toilet paper roll, we could save 423,900 trees.

Sure, we'd still be cutting down 6,681,000 trees each year, but it's a start.

Currently, toilet paper made from 100 percent recycled fiber makes up less than 2 percent of the U.S. market. Compare that to Europe and Latin American, where it makes up about 20 percent of the market.

There are other advantages besides cutting down fewer trees. For example, toilet paper from recycled fiber takes 50 percent less energy to produce and avoids the use of chlorine, which leaves traces of the toxic chemical dioxin.

TP Fun Facts

- The average toilet tear is 5.9 sheets ripped from a roll.

- Forty-four percent of people wipe from front to back.

- Sixty percent look at the paper they've just used.

- Forty-two percent fold their TP, 33 percent crumple, and 8 percent both fold and crumple.

- Six percent wrap their TP around their hands.

- At least 50 percent of people have at one time or another wiped with something other than TP.

- Thirty percent admit to being witnessed by a spouse or partner, waddling with trousers at ankles, eagerly in search of more TP. (Okay, that's just the authors' guess. Have you ever ended up using newspaper, magazines, or your undies? 'Fess up!)

But our favorite reason for using recycled toilet paper comes from Tim Spring, president of recycled TP maker Marcal, who suggests that his toilet paper will lead to—we kid you not—better mental health. "People want to know what happens to the paper they recycle. This will give them *closure* [our italics]."

The Wipe Stuff

While there haven't been any toilet paper revolutions, it's not because companies haven't tried. In 2001, Kimberly-Clark introduced Cottonelle Fresh Rollwipes, the first pre-moistened toilet wipe on a roll. Just what was soaked into those wipes? Kimberly-Clark alluded to comfortable sounding, "mild skin cleansers and emollients" in their press release. Translation? The chemical preservative methylisothiazolinone, aloe, water, salt, glycol propylene, sodium benzoate, Vitamin E, polysorbate 20, malic acid, and lauryl glycoside. All, soooo very comforting! Kimberly-Clark had done a survey that showed that 60 percent of U.S. consumers believed that using a wet wipe was cleaner and more "refreshing" than using dry toilet paper alone. We're guessing that the survey didn't have the follow-up question "Will you be buying said wet wipes?" The answer apparently would have been, "Eh, probably not," because Rollwipes just didn't sell.

What happened? Well, one problem was that Rollwipes came in a special dispenser that had to be connected to an existing toilet paper holder. When a product known for its simplicity states "some assembly required," it is not a big selling point.

Additionally, we have to believe that purchasing wet wipes carries a stigma of personal cleanliness problems. Purchasing it almost seems like an admission that not only does one's shit stink, but it's also apparently messily unmanageable.

❧ DEEP SHIT!

Though they didn't make the big time in the United States, wet wipes have been popular in different countries for a number of years. Kimberly-Clark's Andrex Moist is a popular brand in England. And the Swiss, a people known for their manic tidiness, love a moist cleanup—almost 36 percent of Swiss consumers use premoistened TP. So to fine cheese, watches, alpine vistas, and secret bank accounts, we can now add one more characteristic of Swiss life: a love of the feeling of a wet towelette on one's ass.

As if all that's not enough, it turns out that wet wipes don't degrade as well as regular toilet paper, which can create some stinky problems for septic systems and sketchy plumbing.

Of course we can't fault Kimberly-Clark's logic. When you think about it, we typically don't get cleaner by getting drier. Most of us would prefer not to clean a baby with dry toilet paper alone. Moist wipes help keep a baby's rump and a cleaner's sanity intact.

Rollwipes didn't disappear completely, though. They were just taken off the roll, put in a box, and renamed Cottonelle Fresh Flushable Moist Wipes, once again proving the corporate genius of repackaging.

All this talk of TP omits one important fact: You need to be able to reach around. Sadly, due to injury, deep psychic scars, or physical challenges, not all of us are able to wipe our own asses. And for this group, since porte-cotons and grooms of the stool have long since vanished, American industry has thoughtfully brought us the Comfort Wipe, "the sanitary paper extension arm and holder." As the info-mercial says. "It's as easy to use as a shower brush." We just hope you don't confuse the two. Who would use one? Large people, for starters. "Being a big guy has its disadvantages," notes the hefty lad in the ad.

Back(side) to the Future

What's the future hold for our fibrous old friend? Well, how would you feel about wiping your tuchis with spread-sheets? A Japanese company called Oriental has come up with a product called White Goat, an automatic toilet paper production machine that shreds and compresses office pa-per. The machine, which is about the size of a small mini-van and weighs 1,300 pounds, just needs paper, water, and electricity to work its magic. The Goat can produce a roll of toilet paper in about thirty minutes and requires about forty sheets of used office paper (invoices, reports, harsh employee reviews, etc.) per roll. At a cost of over $100,000, a White Goat might not be in your immediate future, but if you like to roll your own and tend to take private jets to sporting events, you might have found the bathroom equipment of your dreams.

KNOW SHIT!

The French have their own little opportunity to gain knowledge while they leave behind their depoits. Normandy resident Christian Poincheval has designed Petit Lutin toilet paper, which features writing on French culture, geography, news, and current affairs on each sheet. How's it selling? Three times faster than normal TP, according to department store managers.

❦ 7 ❦

IN THE FLUSH

Okay, enough about toilet paper. Let's get to the flushing process itself. It might seem that we are lucky to live in such a hygienic generation. No more pooping off castle walls, no need to walk down the sidewalk in fear that you will be hit flush in the face with bucket-strewn flying feces. And that certainly is, as they say, a plus.

Well, we hate to break it to you, but conditions in your porcelain kingdom might not be as pristine as you think. If you're currently wearing a respirator and scouring the crevices of your bathroom with chlorine, you probably can skip this chapter. If not, brace yourself. And read on.

That's Not Love in the Air

Are you the type of person who puts down the toilet seat when you flush? If not, just know that you might want to become one. Consider the work of Dr. Charles Gerba from the University of Arizona. Dr. Gerba has spent his career studying the germs that inhabit homes, offices, and public spaces. (If you're wondering about his qualifications, just know that he has been called the all-knowing god of bathroom and kitchen germs.)

Using a strobe light flash, Dr. Gerba took photos of a toilet flushing. The results, involving aerosolization, look like a Las Vegas fountain. The good doctor likened this display to a Fourth of July fireworks show. The bad news for us is that the aerosol mist harbors a slew of bacterial bad news. Tests on the mist from public bathrooms have registered positive for the common cold virus, hepatitis A virus, streptococcus, staphylococcus, *E. coli*, and shigella.

KNOW SHIT! ✌

One of the lesser bacterial niches in your bathroom is actually the top of your toilet seat. The bacterial backwater of your bathroom? Your sink, due in part to the accumulations of water, which enables nasty organisms to breed freely after splashdown.

Not yet disgusted enough, the good doctor then went on to conduct tests by placing pieces of gauze in different locations around the bathroom and measuring their bacterial and viral levels after a flush. His studies showed that water droplets in this invisible cloud travel six to eight feet—a bacterial boom, if you like. A microbial mushroom cloud, if you don't.

What do to? Some researchers advise leaving the bathroom immediately after flushing so as not to have the microscopic airborne mist land on you, which is easier said than done. You might want to accomplish this with one hand on a broomstick and the other ready to slam the door behind you. Or flush while simultaneously doing a somersault out of the bacterial blast area.

ꙮ DEEP SHIT!

It's not just your bathroom. There are even dirtier areas in your home and office. For example, for every 49 microbes that you can find per square inch on your toilet seat, you can find a fecal veneer of 1,676 microbes on your computer mouse. That keyboard? 3,295 microbes per square inch. And next time you reach for your phone, think about this: It's plastered with 25,127 germs per square inch.

But even if you get out of the bathroom unscathed by fecal bacteria (which you won't, but hey, it's good to have a goal), that bacterial cloud remains floating. Yep, aerosolization brings new meaning to "Believe me, you don't want to go in there," because it takes at least *two hours* for it to settle. By the way, did you leave your toothbrush by the bathroom sink this morning? Yeah, if you have a medicine cabinet, you might want to keep your toothbrush in there from now on. Or maybe in a Ziploc bag located in a safe-deposit box across town. Whichever is easier.

With all that bacteria floating around your bathroom, it's no wonder that Dr. Gerba has been quoted as saying, "If an alien came from space and studied the bacterial counts, he probably would conclude he should wash his hands in your toilet and crap in your sink."

Let Me See a Show of Hands

What can you do about the fecal bacteria tornado that seemingly spins around you every time you flush the toilet? While it might seem like you are powerless to do anything about it, there are actually some pretty easy solutions.

Wash your hands.

Cleaning your hands is a simple and effective way to combat the spread of germs. (Speaking of which, when was the last time you washed your hands? No, go ahead. Remember to get under the nails. You might want to disinfect this book, too. Thanks.)

❧ DEEP SHIT!

During the seventeenth century, doctors told people that washing would open their pores to the plague. Finally, in 1847, the nicely named Dr. Ignaz Semmelweis discovered that hand washing prevented the spread of disease. He wasn't entirely right, though—he advocated using chlorinated lime solution, which is only one ingredient in chlorine bleach. But it did have the same effect. It wasn't until a few years later that Louis Pasteur's germ theory helped prove that microorganisms were the cause of many diseases that people had a scientific explanation for the need for washing their hands.

KNOW SHIT! ❧

In a 2000 poll, 95 percent of the people surveyed responded that they always wash their hands after using public restrooms. But observers discovered that a third of those using bathrooms did not wash their hands. So while it's good to know that people actually know they *should* wash their hands after using the bathroom, it's a little disheartening to find out that a third of them are dirty, disease-ridden liars.

What About Hand Sanitizer?

Cleaning your hands with alcohol-based hand sanitizer also works. One recent study found that sanitizer is as effective at killing germs as washing hands with soap and water. Hand sanitizer does have one major weakness, though: It can't completely clean hands covered with grime, dirt, or crud. If your hands are covered in mud, all the hand sanitizer is going to do is make them smell like alcohol-scented mud.

KNOW SHIT! ✨

Use a hand sanitizer containing at least 60 percent alcohol, because it is the alcohol that is actually doing the important cleaning, killing the bacteria. Use at least a half teaspoon, or enough that it takes fifteen to twenty seconds to dry.

How About Antibacterial Soap?

So you might be wondering: Since washing hands with soap and water to shed bacteria is so effective, does antibacterial soap do the job even better?

Actually, no.

Antibacterial soap is no better at killing germs than regular soap—and may be worse. Turns out it's the physical act of washing your hands, not the specific variety of soap, that does the hard work of removing and killing germs. What's the "worse" part? According to the Mayo Clinic, antibacterial soap may ultimately prove detrimental, as it can "lead to the development of bacteria . . . resistant to the product's antimicrobial agents—making it harder to kill these germs in the future."

So unless you were planning on helping develop superbacteria that will wipe out life on the planet, you might want to stick with plain old soap. But it's really up to you.

KNOW SHIT!

Does hot water kill more germs than cold water? According to the experts, there's not much difference. Hot water, however, has been shown to be better at removing grease and grime—and it feels better, too!

What if All Employees Don't Wash Their Hands?

Ever wonder why it's so important that employees wash their hands before returning to work, like the sign says?

Simple: Restaurant workers spread foodborne illness through hand contact with the pathogens in their gastrointestinal tract. In layman's terms, they might have shit on their hands. Many diseases like hepatitis A and shigella can be transmitted from person to person through contaminated hands, thanks to inadequate hand washing. It takes only a few particles of hepatitis A to make you ill, and when you realize that a single gram of fecal material can contain 100 million viral particles, you might want to keep an eye on your waiters and waitresses, not to mention the cooks and those bussing the tables. For that matter, keep tabs on the maître d' as well.

So how many employees really do wash their hands?

A study of hand washing sponsored by the U.S. Department of Health and Human Services found that more than half of fast-food industry workers failed to wash their hands properly. And restaurant employees handle about 70 billion meals in the United States each year. You can finish the math. But even if you don't, it's no wonder that about 59 percent of foodborne illness outbreaks are associated with restaurants.

So next time you go out to eat, here's our suggestion: When your waiter hands you the wine list, hose him down with hand sanitizer.

Next Stop:
The Outflow

If you live in a city, or the burbs, the next stop for your dearly departed shit is a sewage treatment plant. Sewage treatment plants take in raw influent, which is anything that goes down the drain from sinks, showers, bathtubs, and toilets, as well as storm-drain runoff. Like, for example, poop. And TP. And food scraps. And that baby alligator that turned out to be not such a great pet after all.

What does sewage treatment do? In short, it magically transforms dirty water into clean water.

⌘ DEEP SHIT!

It's common for sewer workers to find diapers, cell phones, jewelry, feminine hygiene products, live animals, dead animals, and guns in sewage plant intakes. Less commonly found—and thank goodness—are bodies. Though New York City does report finding homeless men and women in the sewers on occasion. And in Düsseldorf, Germany, a troubled marriage came to a head when a woman flushed pieces of her husband down the toilet.

How does it do it? To get things rolling, a sewage system uses as much gravity as possible. So when you flush your toilet, the wastewater flows down a pipe that runs down the street, which then hooks up to progressively larger lines leading to your local sewage treatment plant. Since these systems don't always have the luxury of gravity, pump stations are used when your shit needs to move uphill. When your poop finally reaches a wastewater treatment plant, a huge rake or mesh screen removes anything large enough to clog up the works, such as branches, litter, and mafia figures "accidentally" hit by bread trucks.

After this pretreatment, the waste ends up as three layers: scum, wastewater, and sludge. The scum is siphoned off and the sludge is gathered up and removed. Typically, a primary treatment tank might remove 60 to 65 percent of suspended solids.

Next, the wastewater moves on to secondary treatment. Secondary treatment further breaks down the remaining bits of human and food waste and soaps and detergents into their basic biological ingredients. How does this happen? The waste is literally eaten—by bacteria and protozoa, which munch away to their heart's content. They also bind together with these contaminants to make them easier to remove from the wastewater.

Some treatment plants use a third stage, in which the wastewater (now known to the sewage cognoscenti as effluent) is filtered through sand or allowed to soak in a placid lagoon or wetland, where plants and feeding invertebrates give any remaining bacteria another biological kick in the pants. Then at long last that once putrid, shit-filled water is ready to rejoin the happy world of scenic rivers, lakes, and streams. On its way out the door, chlorine or ultraviolet light is used to disinfect the effluent and zap any remaining bacteria.

Shit in the Streets, Birth Control in the Water

Well, that's how it would work—ideally. Unfortunately, sewage treatment plants have their problems, too. For example, too much storm water runoff can cause a plant to discharge partially treated wastewater back into the environment, which is definitely not an ideal shituation.

✦ DEEP SHIT!

Cities with antiquated combined sewer systems often face overflow problems during periods of heavy rain. Runoff from buildings and streets drain into pipes full of untreated sewage, causing them to overflow. Such is the case in Portland, Oregon, where raw sewage overflows into the Willamette River. In worst-case scenarios, power outages at the Oregon City treatment plant exacerbate the situation. In 2009, 3 million gallons of raw sewage drained into the Willamette in six hours.

Another serious problem? Sewage treatment plants don't remove many chemicals from wastewater. For example, for every liter of Puget Sound water, researchers found four milligrams of artificial vanilla. Now this might seem like a bad thing only for those who prefer chocolate. But it's not just vanilla, as scientists around the world have found trace amounts of everything from sugar and cinnamon to heroin and insecticides to rocket fuel and birth control in public water supplies. Currently, sewage treatment just doesn't filter out substances such as these. Doesn't exactly make you thirsty, does it?

What's the only thing worse than having a malfunctioning sewage treatment plant? How about none at all? It's a situation not uncommon in many of the poorer cities of the world—but would you believe it was also true in Italy's capital, Milan? The capital of Italy was still dumping raw sewage into the Lambro River as recently as a decade ago. Only the threat of a $15-million-a-day fine from the European Union got the Milanese to stop their shit from flowing freely.

The Sludge Report

Remember that sludge that was hauled out of the treatment plant? Wondering where it all goes? Good news: These days most of the pesky stuff is handled pretty wisely. But it wasn't always that way.

Take New York City, for example. Sludge from the Big Apple used to be dumped directly into New York Harbor. In 1924, this had to be stopped, because part of the harbor had actually putrefied. That's right. The harbor started to rot. City officials decided to dump the sludge, instead, twelve miles out in the ocean. When that site became too contaminated, the sludge was hauled another ninety-four miles out to sea.

But it turned out that out of sight wasn't exactly out of mind. In 1992, dead fish, syringes, and toxic metals all started washing up on New Jersey beaches, and ocean dumping had to be stopped. What's happened since then? For years, the sludge was actually loaded onto a line of red railcars and dumped on a 128,000-acre ranch in—get ready for this—Sierra Blanca, *Texas.* Later, New York paid a fertilizer company to take the 1,200 daily tons of sludge. To save money, the city later cancelled the deal and dumped the sludge directly into landfills. At last check, New York was looking for ways to make cold cash out of its warm shit, and was searching for a company willing to turn its heaps of sludge into heat and power.

Sludge has come a long way. These days much of it is treated to reduce the amount of pathogens and becomes the much more friendly-sounding biosolids, which are then used as fertilizer or burned for energy. But sludge remains a pesky problem. Even treated biosolids can contain PCBs, dioxin, and flame retardants—not exactly what you want your tomatoes grown in, but it's probably better than having a rotting harbor.

Small-Town Shit

If you live in the burbs or in the sticks, like a quarter of the country, the final resting place for your poop is actually just outside your door: your septic system.

The septic system was invented in the 1860s in France by Jean-Louis Mouras. Mouras, clearly ahead of his time when it comes both marketing and shit, called his invention *la vidangeuse automatique*, or "the automatic cleaning lady."

KNOW SHIT!

It has been said that Mouras thought up his septic system, built it—then buried it. After a dozen years of using it, he dug it up and found out that it worked. Chalk up a victory for lazy science!

Before your septic system can do its thing, however, your shit first has to get there. How does that happen? Well, this might seem a bit surprising, but the guiding force in most septic systems is old-fashioned gravity. (Besides, who wants to live downhill from his [or her] shit?)

Septic systems are amazingly simple. Think of a septic system as an incredibly foul-tasting layered birthday cake. Waste flows out to the septic tank and eventually forms three layers. Poop solids float to the bottom, forming a sludge layer, gray water moves to the middle, and oil and grease float to the surface to form a scum layer.

Bacteria helps to break down the waste into those layers. And where does the bacteria come from? It comes from you! Remember that gut flora that helps break food down into poop? It keeps working long after it has escaped from your colon.

As new waste flows into the tank, the liquid shit water that's been eaten by bacteria flows out of the septic tank. That middle layer of water then flows into a buried set of small pipes, called a leach or drain field. The heavy sludge, however, gets left behind.

KNOW SHIT!

Is the grass really greener over the septic tank? Yes, and here's why. As the wastewater travels through the leach field and into the ground, microbes remove bacteria and viruses, purifying the water. One of the by-products? Nutrients that fertilize the ground.

As for the sludge layer, every couple of years it needs to be pumped out. And unless your local pumper is shadily dumping it in his neighbor's pool, it's treated just like big city sludge and is either processed at a wastewater plant or treated and sold as biosolids—where it just might end up being spread on your local farm.

Sometimes Simple Things Can Be Complicated

It's true that septic systems are amazingly simple. But it's also true that even simple things can fail. And when they do, the results can be, well, dramatic. Here are four ways septic systems commonly fail and the nasty results:

Failure 1: Too Much Shit

Take, for example, putting in too much shit. It might seem like a great money-saving idea to have that wedding in your backyard, but when eighty guests all poop on the same day, the bride might actually step in the groom's shit as it surfaces from a clogged leach field.

Failure 2: The Pet Funeral

Because septic systems are made just for poop, pee, and water, they can clog when things like tampons, condoms, and deceased guinea pigs are flushed down the drain. The result? Shit will back up . . . and up . . . and up. Until it comes out the first opening it can find, which in many houses can be the kitchen sink.

Failure 3: Killing Your Septic System

Thanks to the bacteria in the septic tank, septic systems are literally alive. And they, too, can be killed—by chemicals, gasoline, pesticides, antifreeze, and paint that get poured down the drain by not-so-bright homeowners. And when the bugs die, the shit piles up. And up—and now you know how that ends.

Failure 4: The Exploding Septic System

As if all of these problems weren't annoying enough, your septic system has one last trick: It can explode in a hail of high-velocity shit. How does your septic system turn into a bomb? As part of the process of breaking down the waste, methane gas is produced. Methane is explosive unless it is properly vented. If it's not, as with some of the earliest attempts at septic systems, you've got a highly unstable shit-bomb situation on your hands. How did septic designers and morose homeowners discover this? You guessed it! The hard way.

From splintered toilet paper to the fecal veneer on your computer monitor to exploding septic systems, cleaning up just isn't as tidy and simple as it might seem at first wipe. But if you think that's a long, strange story, grab your passport, take a deep breath, and calm your colon. You're about to experience a road trip unlike any other: a shit-filled journey around the world!

8

THE WONDERFUL
WORLD OF POO

What do nomads in the Sahel region of Africa, Parisian pastry chefs, and Panamanian Kuna Indians have in common? Why, shit, of course! A brown biological bond, our shit ties those of us in North America with our brothers and sisters in poop on vastly different shores. While pooping is a necessity, our diverse cultures regard, acknowledge, and occasionally feel terrible shame about our daily urge to purge in vastly different ways. If you've assumed that the rest of the world shits like you do—seated in private on a porcelain throne, flushing with water that is as clean as the stuff you drink—well, you're about to snap out of your hygienic reverie. And then there's the post-poop cleanup. You think toilet paper is universal? You're about to learn to clean your bum all over again.

Ready for a Magical Shittery Tour, from the fecal phobic to the fecal philiac? Step right up! (Actually, you might want to watch where you step, but more on that in a moment.)

Toilet Tours—Asia, Ltd.

Yes, thanks mostly to geographic conditions and economic disparities, bathroom etiquette and toilet styles around the world do vary. And nowhere is it more different from North America than in Asia, where toilets range from a simple pit in the ground to the most opulent on earth. For most Asians, pooping still means squatting over an open hole usually in a humid room or building. Turkey and the Indian subcontinent feature the classic squat toilet, a porcelain tray recessed into the floor with footrests on either side.

ᴥᴥᴥ DEEP SHIT!

Culturally confused about how best to poop in India? Engineers in that country have come to the rescue! After locals kept standing on the rims or seats of toilet bowls and breaking the seats, they devised a dual-culture toilet. The seat can be lowered for those preferring a Western-style toilet or raised to reveal two porcelain footprints for those favoring the squatting position.

Thailand's toilets, on the other hand, consist of a small raised porcelain pedestal with footrests. The downside?

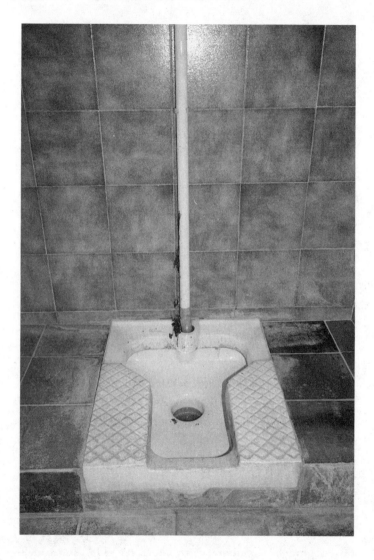

This potty requires delicate balance to avoid unseemly mishaps or "the most unforgettable vacation moment ever." And over in Japan, birthplace of the high-tech toilet, public facilities still feature squats—elongated floor slots with small covers to catch any splashing.

While they may not agree on the best kind of toilets, Asians can agree that the preferred wipe comes with water. Consequently, you can count on the floor in the bathroom always being wet. Toilet paper is available, though if it's used at all, it's used to dry rather than cleanse. Besides, for most Asians, the cost of TP is prohibitive. And what's the point, anyway? Septic systems can't handle the paper and it rapidly fills up pit holes.

Getting Wet

While our tour is still in Asia, let's take a moment and consider the post-poop cleanup. How many of us have ever considered wiping our butts with anything other than triple-ply lavender-lotioned toilet paper? Anything else just seems unsanitary and a little abhorrent, right? Not according to most of the world—or scientific studies, for that matter. In fact, washing one's ass after pooping not only dates back thousands of years but also is promoted by certain religious laws. Hindus, for example, were so vested in washing their butts after pooping that they initially refused to believe that Europeans wiped their butts with paper.

DEEP SHIT!

Many believe that thorough butt cleansing is achievable only by washing after each poop. Western-style dry wiping, it turns out, leaves behind fecal residue. In fact, a British study of men's underpants revealed fecal contamination ranging from colored stains to visible fecal flecks. Perhaps warm bidet water and public ridicule has encouraged these men to change their cleanup habits. Still, it hasn't dissuaded the Brits from tossing some advice in our direction. "You don't wipe, you blot!"

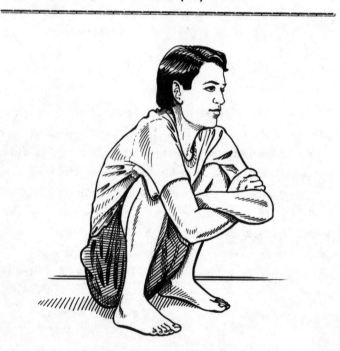

Just how does one clean up with water? Many Asian bathrooms are outfitted with a small plastic bucket and a trough
full of water or a small tap. While India is a country of buckets, Thailand is a country of hoses. In either case, you can be
sure of one thing—if there is a faucet, it is likely to leak. The
plastic bucket and short hose, or bum gun, aren't there to
clean the bowl, either. Think of them as a do-it-yourself
bidet. Just point the nozzle toward your sphincter and turn
the knob! (Did you just try this at home? Did you just yelp?
We may have forgotten to tell you to test the pressure of the
hose first before aiming it at any bodily orifices. Sorry.)

KNOW SHIT! ❧

**Visiting a private home in Japan? Don't forget to change out of
regular shoes into a pair of house shoes and then, before entering
the bathroom, replace the house shoes with plastic bathroom
slippers.**

But what about post-poop cleansing in areas where water
is scarce? Simple! Users skip the water, go left (see page
172), and then smear their shit-encrusted hand across any
available surface—decorating walls, ceilings, and floors in
the process. Once dry, fecal patties make excellent message

boards (with the message obviously being "There is no toilet paper in this restroom."), or so we're told. Here's a disturbing fact: Tic-tac-toe grids have been found etched into dried fecal walls. While we realize that all cultures are different, we have a hard time believing there are any winners in a game of shit-tac-toe.

Go Left, Young Man

The sorry fact is, we in the paper culture may not be using the most effective medium for cleansing our asses. Other parts of the world believe that there is a better way—using your left hand and going left. A time-honored tradition, going left is actually split into two camps: the dry cleaners and the wet wipers. A dry cleaner simply uses a dry left hand to digitally remove any poop particles. (Be careful to avoid lodging any of those solids under your fingernails!) With the right hand, the dry leftie pours water over the left hand, rinsing off the particles. (Repeat as necessary, just like shampooing!) In contrast, the wet wiper uses his right hand to pour water over his bum while scrubbing with his left. Wet wiping occurs in homes, in hedges, and on train tracks. It's the cleanup of choice of the open defecator—a man or woman scuttling about carrying a small plastic pitcher, searching for privacy in rural villages and overpopulated slums alike.

Top Three Open Defecation Nations

1. China, 670 million
2. India, 560 million
3. Indonesia, 70 million

We can't leave Asia without offering our heartfelt congratulations to the little Nepali village of Puma, in the Lamjung region. They recently went open defecation free as part of International Sanitation Week. Over five hundred residents and dignitaries attended the celebration, which included mothers holding signboards displaying the new rules.

They seem to be:

· Defecating in the open is disgusting and unhealthy.

· I shall not defecate in the open.

· I will use a latrine at all times.

· I will practice good hygiene.

Other Nepalese communities have taken things a step further, engaging the community in the shameful walk, showing people the places they defecate openly and organizing a feces-flagging exercise, where the community places paper flags on feces lying around. The end goal? The community feels ashamed and disgusted by its open defecation practice!

❧❧❧ DEEP SHIT!

Just finished pooping and realized there's no TP within scuttling reach? Don't panic. It's time to go left! In the squatting position, take the little hose or water pitcher with your right hand and aim or pour water over your bum while with the left hand (fingers extended with tips pulled back) wiping until clean. Then get another scoop of water and pour fresh water over your left hand until clean. (This may take a very, very long time.) Use the right hand for eating, shaking hands, or just about anything else other than wiping your rear.

Toilet Tours—South America, Ltd.

Continuing on our global toilet trot, let's take brief stop in South America to examine their *baños* and *servicios públicos*. Generally speaking, toilets are more homogeneous than language on this continent. They're readily available and pretty well maintained. North American dry wipers will be glad to know that many of the toilets are even stocked with TP of some kind.

✤✦✤ DEEP SHIT!

Traveling in South America and need to poop? Keep your eyes peeled for pay-to-access *servicios públicos*. A few *pesos* will grant you access to a toilet that varies from a hole in the ground to a porcelain flush toilet. Many of these public toilets are located on private land, and a family member tends to the toilet during the day to supplement the family income.

In remote corners of South America, toilets adapt to the local environment. High on the Andean plateau, adobe outhouses made of local bricks dot the Cordillera mountain range. In the Bolivian Altiplano region, toilets are carved out of de-thorned cacti, the only material available in this dry landscape, and strategically positioned over holes. Meanwhile, on the Panamanian coast, the Kuna Indians have erected toilets overhanging the ocean. Above a picturesque turquoise sea, these *servicios* stand on stilts and are reachable only by walking over rickety narrow planks.

Toilet Tours—Africa, Ltd.

South America may have its shit together, but across the Atlantic, it's a study in contrasts. Toilets—or the lack thereof—highlight the huge economic disparities of Africa. For some, sanitation and waste disposal facilities still linger in the dark ages. Nomadic cultures across the continent poop in the open while running down antelope just as they did thousands of years ago. Meanwhile, trendy urbanites frequenting Johannesburg nightclubs find themselves pooping into sleek chrome receptacles. Sad but true: The continent on which man took his first satisfying shit still searches for poop equity.

KNOW SHIT!

Outhouse holes in sub-Saharan Africa are deep—really deep. In many places around the globe, the soil is too rocky to effectively dig deep pits; outhouse pits are usually an average of five to eight feet deep. But in sub-Saharan Africa, pits go way deep—often to a depth of forty feet, which means they have the added benefit of being slow to fill.

Africa's cultural and geographic diversity is reflected in the places people poop. Across the northern part of the continent, classic Turkish-style squat toilets prevail. In the southern part of the continent, Africans prefer seated toilets; the thrones are usually constructed of wood or molded out of local clay and stone. But across rural Africa, villagers rely on outhouses constructed of corrugated metal or local mud bricks for a little privacy. It's the style to use hinge-less, colorful doors propped against the entrance to the outhouse.

KNOW SHIT! 🌿

In our travels around the world, there's one toilet we've so far neglected to check out . . . the one in your local prison. If your local jailhouse was built more than a century ago, it might not even have potties in the cell. In that case, prisoners poop into buckets, and morning chores feature a sordid routine called slopping out. Modern pens, on the other hand, have semi-stalls with short sidewalls and no door, so guards can keep one eye on the dumping jailbird. At home in the cell, prisoners use one-piece, built-in stainless units that include a sink and toilet—sans seat since, of course, anything that's not nailed down might just end up being used as a cudgel or for a suicide. (And if you're thinking about killing yourself by slamming a stainless-steel toilet seat down on your head, life really has hit rock bottom.)

Toilet Tours—Europe, Ltd.

How different can things be in Europe, a continent noted for its sophistication, fine wines, and spotless city sidewalks? *Very* different. Europe, it turns out, sports a diverse array of toilets, from fully automated self-cleaning stainless-steel gems to some of the stinkiest, scariest holes on the globe. Luckily, we can split the continent by its east-west axis—a great toilet divide, as it were. North of Italy, bathrooms are bountiful and feature seated toilets; south of the border (that includes you, Provence), toilets are seen as more of a bare necessity. They're infrequent and are often squat-only.

❧ DEEP SHIT!

The city of Paris is undergoing a revival in public restrooms. Once known for having some of the worst public facilities, Paris now has new self-cleaning Sanisettes popping up all over the city. New models use rainwater to flush, and even feature skylights! You'd better use them, too—because Paris's Bad Behavior Brigade can slap you with a $600 fine for relieving yourself in public.

There's another difference between northern Europe and southern, too: whether you care to inspect your poo. Up in Germany, the toilet shelves are perfect for shit analysis—and also give users a chance to admire ingenious German engineering. The Italians, however, have decided to let go and have no need to linger over their poo. As a result, Italian bowls are steep and deep, with only a couple of inches of water in the very bottom, denying the user a chance to thoroughly inspect her handiwork. There's one stinky problem with this design, though: A misaimed poo will tumble down the sides of the waterless bowl, leaving a smear so horrible it just might put you off your pasta.

One feature is common across the continent, though: You've got to pay to poop, and you never know what you'll find lurking inside. Some toilets are coin operated, but many feature a toilet attendant who will also dispense TP if there's none in the stalls. And what's that seemingly extra urinal next to the toilet? It's a bidet.

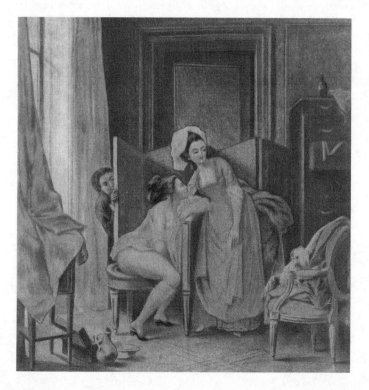

That's right. No need to look away. The bidet has long been unjustly associated with kinky European sex habits and loose women. *Mais non!* The bidet is, according to Europeans, just another cultural divide between *us* and *them* (the United States being the *them* in this case) and one that leaves their nether regions superiorly clean. It's difficult for us to grasp why Europeans install a child-size sink into closet-sized bathrooms while leaving little room for the shower—until, that is, you've given yourself a first-degree burn with recycled toilet paper or your mother has complained about the skid marks in your shorts in front of your friends.

KNOW SHIT! ❧

Need a little assistance? Toilet attendants are called madame pipi in France or Klofrau in Germany. And it seems as if this is a profession dominated by women in these countries, as you're hard pressed to find a monsieur pipi or an Herr Klomann.

Finally, a word of warning for women who are grabbing their passports and jetting off to Europe. Should you venture out to enjoy the nightlife with the locals, you might have to get a bit more personal than you'd prefer. If you're headed to the bathroom, chances are you'll first have to walk by a row of urinals in the common area before you

World's Worst Toilets*

1. China
2. India
3. France
4. Italy

5. Thailand
6. Egypt
7. Turkey
8. Mexico

*As rated by the tourists who have used them, according to the Titanic Awards.

reach the unisex stalls. And unless you can get yourself through that tiny little window, you're going to have to walk past them when you leave.

The Great Poo Divide

Consider this sad fact: *Forty percent of the world's population does not have proper human waste disposal facilities.* In India, for example, 700 million people are forced to defecate in the open. In some Delhi slums, 480,000 families have access to only 270 toilets. And it doesn't get any better in Africa. In one Nairobi slum, 40,000 people share 10 pit latrines.

With a lot more asses than toilets, people predictably take matters into their own hands. In crowded cities without the hope of privacy or government solutions, slum residents have developed the flying toilet. One simply defecates into the ubiquitous plastic bag, waits for nightfall, and then hurls the bag onto the nearest rooftop or alley. If that sounds like a bad idea, consider that visiting the few available public toilets is probably much more hazardous to your health. In Ghana, for example, the walls of public toilets often are smeared with feces from floor to ceiling, even though there's an attendant at the ready to sell you toilet paper. And who can blame them? Money's tight, and that TP—well, it's really just pages torn from newspapers. Smearing your fecal fingers is effective and certainly cheaper.

KNOW SHIT!

Public toilets are a rare find worldwide. School toilets in developing countries are often locked or never cleaned. UNICEF estimates that poor sanitation alone results in a 30 percent dropout rate. In Tanzania, India, and Bangladesh, school enrollment increased by 15 percent when schools installed and maintained decent toilets.

In rapidly growing urban areas, barrios, and slums, private toilets are rare and communal toilets are overcrowded and, as a result, overflowing. So city residents poop as their ancestors did. The only problem? They're no longer in the bush and there are a lot more people. On a typical dawn hour in Nepal's capital Kathmandu, urbanites scuttle about the shrubbery in parks, retreat into dark alleyways, and stride confidently toward local waterways. Alongside their morning offerings of marigolds and rice to the gods, the Nepalese are leaving different offerings—all which eventually find their way to the holy Bagmati River. Sadly, the resultant illnesses such as diarrhea, typhoid, and cholera are often lethal. Those who are fortunate enough to have their homes connected to municipal sewage lines still have their karma to worry about: Those drains head right to the city's holy rivers, making the entire city sick. During monsoon season, streets and sewers overflow, creating rivulets with brown shapeless masses bobbing their way to the holy Bagmati and Vishnumati rivers.

KNOW SHIT!

In the Mekong River Delta, the Vietnamese conduct their business in overhung toilets, shacks erected over the river delta and ponds. Daily deposits feed fish, bringing a whole new disturbing meaning to *bottom feeders*.

Traveling with Your Shit

Whether you're passing through Latin America, Asia, or Europe, one thing's for sure: You're about to experience many firsts: your first bidet, your first opportunity to go left (if you choose to attempt it), your first squat. You get the picture—toilet etiquette sure isn't anything like what you've experienced on your home throne. And for better or worse, you're going to be depositing shit along the way. Thankfully, though, you now know how to handle that funny short hose by the toilet, the plastic bucket and cup— even that oddly low sink with the spray nozzle in which you once tried to wash your hands.

But, a few shitty little conundra might still catch you with your pants down. Fortunately, we've prepared these Poo Travel Tips. (Lonely Planet, eat your colon out!)

Poo Tip 1: If you're a looker, don't panic if you don't recognize your poo while you're abroad. Its color, shape, and consistency will change—sometimes dramatically. Mentally prepare yourself for a different kind of culture shock.

Poo Tip 2: In Europe, you'll find every kind of toilet, from stainless-steel self-cleaning stalls to Turkish squat toilets. And when it comes to bidding adieu, anything flies. So before you give up and leave your shit stewing, make sure you've pushed, pulled, touched, turned, cranked, and stomped on every knob, sensor, and pull cord in the joint. The flushing mechanism is in there somewhere; you just gotta find it.

Poo Tip 3: Should you find yourself traveling through Latin America, pack your own TP or be prepared to fork over some dinero for *papel higiénico*. A word of warning about the local paper: It's thin, so go easy or your fingers might change color, and not in a good way, either. Oh, and one other thing: Never, ever, flush the TP—it goes in the wastebasket. But you probably already figured that out from the flies buzzing over the trash cans as well as the telltale olfactory clues, didn't you?

Poo Tip 4: If your ass is parked in an Italian, French, or Spanish toilet, we hope you remembered to bring in the TP. It's in the hall. What, you forgot? Let's hope you don't get spotted doing the trou-down shuffle, or you'll definitely have some explaining to do. Crazy American! And if you're Canadian, this is one of those good times to claim to be American. There's no reason to drag your beautiful country into this.

Poo Tip 5: Carry your own personal bidet in your bag—*just in case*. All you need is a sports water bottle. One that you will remember never, ever to drink from again.

Poo Tip 6: Find yourself in Italy or Germany, where your poo can leave skid marks on poop shelves so extensive it looks like you were hanging from a pipe on the ceiling when you jettisoned your poop? Look around. You should find a little rubber toilet brush just for de-smearing purposes.

Poo Tip 7: Be ready to improvise. If you are ill prepared, realize that you might be required to go left. Who knows, maybe you'll even enjoy it. If not, you may have to wipe with a sock or headband if circumstances dictate. If both possibilities don't sound like your cup of tea, you might want to consider trading Bangkok for Brussels.

Poo Tip 8: Try the bidet. Vacations are a great time to experience something new. Forget the stereotype that bidets are for the elderly or the hemorrhoid prone or for post-sex ablutions. They're for *everyone*! Besides, they're in 97 percent of Italian and French bathrooms, so you can't avoid them. Convince yourself that warm water will refresh and rejuvenate your fundaments.

Poo Tip 9: There is no tip 9. Which, is our way of saying that sometimes you're just plain out of luck. Which, conveniently, leads us to our next section: crapping your pants.

On Soiling One's Pants

There's one thing we haven't yet told you about pooping abroad. If the locale is exotic enough, chances are good that at some point you're going to suffer from explosive liquefied shit due to the change in diet or the unfamiliar bugs lurking in your food (but try not to let that keep you from enjoying a delicious street samosa in New Delhi). And not just your run-of-the-ass diarrhea, as we've discussed earlier. We're talking about a gooey shit storm so bad, it begins almost at the point of discharge, with a shooting peristaltic wave strong enough to hose the interior of whatever room, alley, or ditch you have hidden yourself away in.

✕⊙⊙ DEEP SHIT!

Director Danny Boyle reveals that the realistic shit in that memorable cesspit dive scene from *Slumdog Millionaire* actually consisted of . . . peanut butter and chocolate. Will Häagen-Dazs's Chocolate Peanut Butter ice cream ever taste the same again?

If the force of the explosive diarrhea hasn't knocked you against a wall and left you unconscious, you may notice something intriguing. That liquid shit your butt just expelled? It's more of a butternut squash color than a chocolate brown. And this, dear reader, is the universal color and consistency of shit on the Indian subcontinent. From the rice paddies of Jakarta to the dark urban street corners of Dhaka, Bangladesh, this liquefied shit covers the landscape in hues of curry, turmeric, and chili; one misstep in this greasy sidewalk mess can send you sliding out of your flip-flops and leave you slathered in caramel brown.

International Careers in Shit

Forgot your water jug? Left your shreds of newspaper at home? Run out of corncobs? Never fear. In many developing countries, it's customary for toilets to be staffed, usually

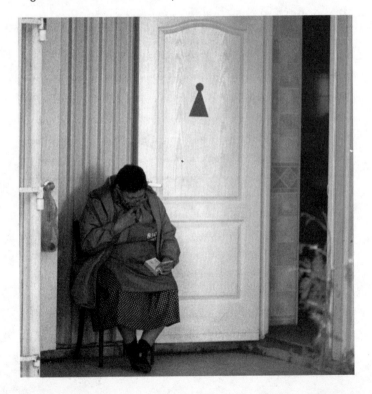

by women or children who collect a small fee. For a pittance
you might also get a few shards of scratchy wiping material.
In the U.K., on the other hand, things are often a bit more
upscale. Toilet attendants await the user with paper towels,
cologne, and hand lotion, and are concerned more with
their tip than your privacy. The attendant trend seems to be
spreading, too, as sexy nightclubs and high-end restaurants
are getting in on the act, hoping that the presence of an
homme de la toilette will help justify the evening's tab in the eyes
of their customers.

Throughout history, there have always been people whose
jobs involved cleaning up other people's messes. Perhaps
the most infamous of these lowly workers are India's Safai
Karamchari, who have made an ancestral profession out of
it—because, unfortunately for them, they're born into it.
Among the scheduled castes with other underclass groups,
these shit wallahs are employed by companies, towns,
railways—even armies. The job, of course, is always the
same: Scrape shit off the streets and clean out the latrines.

How do they do it? Shit wallahs use pieces of scrap metal
to carefully scrape poop into baskets and then carry the
waste away on their heads and shoulders. It's risky business.
Unfortunately, the pay is shit, too—often the Safai Karamchari are compensated for their poop hauling with leftover
chapatis and other food scraps.

Too bad for the shit wallahs that they weren't born in
China, where they might at least make a profit. Many

Shanghai residents still use chamber pots, though the traditional wooden carts of shit collectors have finally been replaced by municipal trucks.

One particularly famous Chinese shit collector of yore was Sister Ah Gui, aka Fen Huang Hou, the shit queen. She lived from 1863 to 1953 and, as boss of all the shit collectors, was rumored to have earned the equivalent of $12,000 a month!

KNOW SHIT! ✿

Chinese shit haulers come by in the early morning hours, driving wooden carts through the streets and shouting, "Leaving! Won't be back!"

But perhaps the most dedicated of shit cleaners are the Tanzanian pit emptiers, known locally as *kutapisha*, who manually empty entire pits through a complex decanting method. To access the pit, the *kutapisha* must first destroy the squatting slab. Then they add about ten pounds of salt to the latrine to break up any solids. They wait two days before returning with a can of kerosene, which they pour into the liquid muck to mask the smell. The fecal slurry is then dug out with simple hand tools like spades and shovels and transferred into a storage pit, barrels, or a desludging vehicle, while the old pit is refurbished with a new concrete slab. Why go through all this trouble? Unfortunately, there's simply no room in crowded settlements to relocate pit toilets. The city of Durban, South Africa, empties its 100,000 pit toilets every five years. That's 20,000 toilets a year in a city where a high percentage of pit sites are in hilly, densely settled areas inaccessible to vehicles.

KNOW SHIT! ✍

In Bangkok, women drive brightly colored mobile toilet trucks to neighborhoods without toilets or to festivals and public squares. These women live in the cabs of their trucks, some replete with Buddhist shrines and TVs.

Seas of Shit, Mountains of Fertilizer

While the Western world has spent centuries trying to bury its shit, one country has been busy turning it into gold: China. For centuries, the Chinese have been collecting, composting, and marketing crap other than their usual plastic kind. Shit-laden fields, the Chinese concluded, yielded tastier, bigger, healthier fruits and vegetables. In fact, one province was so intent on capitalizing on its grossest national product, it mounted a "Seas of Shit, Mountains of Fertilizer" campaign.

KNOW SHIT! ❧

Ninety percent of China's human shit is biologically treated to remove pathogens, filtered, and then spread on fields—and one person's annual poop can fertilize 885 square feet. All told, that's a lot of shit-grown bean sprouts!

Such rear-centric thinking continues today. In fact, China's now the world leader in tapping collective asses for power. Over 15 million families convert human biogas into cooking fuel and electricity. It's not as simple as connecting your butt to your burner, but it is pretty straightforward. Your shit goes into a digester, where microorganisms break down your poop into sugars and acids. These are digested further to release flammable methane gas that helps cook the next mung-bean-based dinner. And the cycle repeats.

KNOW SHIT! ❧

The shit-power arms race is on—and little Nepal is winning! The mountain kingdom has more digesters per capita than China. Unlike China, though, Nepal's digesters are powered by animal dung.

It's a diverse world of shit out there, no doubt about that. A solitary poop can start with anything from pad thai to peach cobbler, and can find itself lying alone on a shit shelf in a German toilet or in a basket atop the head of a third-generation shit wallah in Delhi. And while cultural differences sometimes lead to misunderstandings, we hope this little fecal world tour has led instead to a greater appreciation. Even if you don't suddenly feel closer to your fellow pooper around the globe, look on the bright side: At least now when you see that hose sitting next to the squat toilet on your trip overseas, you can reach for it with the same easy confidence as someone who's gone left his whole life! (And then you can spend the rest of your vacation literally washing your hands of the whole business.)

✿ DEEP SHIT!

Looking for employment? A toilet in Musiri, India, pays its "donors." This first-of-its-kind pooper turns both shit and urine into fertilizer for the local banana crop. How's the pay? Don't quit your day job. The most you stand to make is twelve cents a month.

❧ 9 ☙

THIS SHIT HAS A FUTURE

Shit's come a long way over the centuries, from being unceremoniously dropped on the savannah to being sucked into NASA's ultra-high-tech zero-gravity waste collection system. How will our poops greet the world in the centuries to come? And might they even be processed a bit, well, *differently*? Let's look into our magic ceramic bowl and check out a few pooply trends for the future.

Trend 1: Artificial Digestion

We have to admit that we're a little disappointed. We're into the twenty-first century and not yet at the point where we can order artificial organs from the Internet. Scientists at Britain's Institute of Food Research are hard at work on it, though! They've built the world's first entirely artificial stomach.

Created to help study how the stomach works, the robo-stomach helps researchers study and develop supernutrients and obesity-fighting foods. But before we go putting this robo-tummy in patients, there are still a few kinks that need to be worked out. Like the size, for example, which is about the same as a desktop computer. And the cost, a princely $1.8 million. Both of which are, frankly, a little tough to swallow.

KNOW SHIT!

The Institute of Food Research's artificial stomach is made of special plastics and metals to survive stomach acids and is so realistic that it can even vomit!

And while there hasn't been a lot of progress on other poop-related organs, scientists have built something rather curious for the end of the line for those unfortunate few suffering from fecal incontinence: the Acticon Neosphincter, which simulates the function of the anal sphincter muscle. A fluid-filled device, the Neosphincter is implanted in the body and can be inflated to maintain bowel control. It's not an ideal solution, but when you can't control

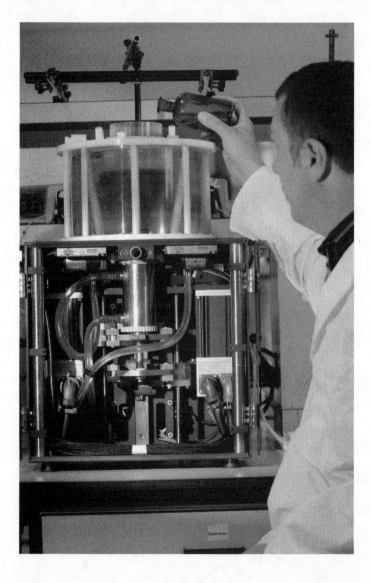

how or when shit comes out of your body, you'll take what you can get.

Trend 2: Eco-Friendly Pooping

Whether we like it or not, our old friend the porcelain throne is being seriously rethought. Toilets are being combined with other bathroom functions, becoming more eco-friendly, and integrating some extremely high-tech poop-related applications. So who's the heir to the throne? Have a seat, and we'll look at some of the latest developments.

✂◦◦ DEEP SHIT!

Kohler's Purist Hatbox toilet is totally tankless and uses a tiny electric pump to help flush out the bowl after use. Coming in for a night landing? Try the Fountainhead edition, a tankless toilet featuring a heated seat and integrated bowl lighting.

One of the biggest environmental drawbacks to modern pooping is the enormous use of water. Toilet designers are hard at work trying to rethink flushing all that H_2O. Caroma's Profile Smart toilet, for example, looks like the unlikely union of a sink and a toilet, but it actually reflects some pretty clever thinking. After flushing, the water that fills up the toilet tank runs through the sink. You can wash your hands and the used water is repurposed for the next flush. Thankfully, Caroma got the sequence correct, so poopers weren't washing up with the toilet outflow.

Meanwhile, Designer Dang Jinwei has come up with the water-saving Home Core integrated toilet, a compact, resource-efficient combination sink/vanity mirror/storage toilet, kind of like a bathroom Swiss Army knife, but without the sharp bits.

Far be it from us to flush somebody's integrated toilet down the bad-idea pipe, but it does seem as though, with so many combinations and arrangements available, mistakes could be made. Terrible, terrible mistakes. It's three in the morning and you're barely awake. Did you just accidently shit in a drawer?

Trend 3: Super High-Tech Toilets— We're Not in Kansas Anymore, Toto

Toto—already the maker of the most complicated toilets in the world—are not resting on their buttocks. They're hard at work designing their latest version of the intelligent toilet. Now, *intelligent* might be overrating their ceramic offspring a bit, but the prototype is definitely one smart-ass toilet. Along with all the usual Toto bells and whistles, such as a heated seat, relaxing music, armrests, and soft-closing lids, this futuristic toilet can measure the blood sugar in one's urine and calculate one's blood pressure, body temperature, and weight. This personal information can be sent to your computer and compared to your past records. It might even let your doctor know that you're running a fever. All of this is great, but we have to imagine the unnerving day in the future when the only email in your inbox is from your toilet—and it's telling you it's time to drop a few pounds.

❧ DEEP SHIT!

One area where the Toto toilet has to catch up is social networking. Computer programmer Seth Hardy made his toilet the first rest stop on the information superhighway when he set it up to send out a message on Twitter every time it was flushed. Obviously he had too much time on his hands, and so did anybody else who was following his ass's status updates.

Is it too far-fetched to think that at some time in the relatively close future we'll be able to get so much information from our toilets, we'll be bragging about them at parties? We foresee a day when people use toilet stats as a cocktail party conversation starter, as in, "Nice toilet you have there. I just weighed in at one pound, two ounces. You?"

Trend 4: Processing Your Poop at Home

"What do we do with *all that poop*?" is one of the great poop questions of the future.

Composting toilets just might be the answer. Sure,

they've been on the market since the alternative movement in the Sixties, but vast improvements now make them an option for every home. They take up about the same space as a typical flush toilet, but use little or no water to flush and don't have a connection to a septic or sewer system. Instead, waste is stored in a compartment under the toilet or goes to a special chamber to compost. And the old odor issues have since been addressed with fans for aeration and a fresh layer of sawdust or peat moss post-use. So you no longer need to spray a bottle of patchouli after each use.

DEEP SHIT!

The future is so bright, we've gotta wear shades! There are more than two dozen shit-related iPhone apps available. They include the Poo Log, which helps you catalog and understand your daily dumps, and Poop the World, to socially share the latest news on your fresh dump. Then there's Poop! for those moments when you desperately need to find a public toilet, and even Butt Muffler, which produces a variety of household noises to mask even your noisiest of farts.

Composting toilets now vary from a simple twin-chamber design in which waste composts in one chamber while the other fills, to mechanized systems where rotating tines mix the waste and temperature and moisture probes control electronic systems. But they all carry out the same process of decomposition in the presence of aerobic decomposers who convert the waste into valuable nutrient-rich compost.

A new twist in the world of composting toilets is the Envirolet FlushSmart VF vacuum flush. While it does use water, it uses just a fifth of a liter, compared to a typical toilet, which can use up to thirteen liters. A vacuum system zips your poop off to a composting tank and out of olfactory range.

Trend 5: Poo Power!

What if all that poop could be power instead? Turning shit into shining light is truly the holy grail of the poop world. Hard at work on that effort is the British company SEaB Energy, who has developed the MuckBuster, a self-contained anaerobic digester. Poop goes in, and four weeks later, biogas and fertilizer come out. Pretty neat, huh?

We have only two not-so-minor complaints. There's the twenty-foot shipping container, which is just a bit too big to fit between the TP roll and the plunger. There's also the matter of the couple of hundred liters of waste a day that's needed to make the MuckBuster work. We don't want to be sticks in the muck, but unless you can bring the delicate topic of shit up at your next neighborhood association meeting, the MuckBuster might not be your ideal home solution.

Then there's Virginia Gardiner's LooWatt, a toilet intended to fill an important global need. According to Gardiner, 2.6 billion people around the world don't have access to toilet facilities. That's more than a third of the population of the planet. The LooWatt is a very simple closed system. Use the LooWatt, then take the collected waste to a nearby biodigester processing facility, which then turns the waste into methane. For your effort, you walk away with a canister of methane fuel to cook your food . . . which eventually leads you full circle, back to the LooWatt.

KNOW SHIT! ✿

Taking the reuse of shit concept one step further than anyone else, the LooWatt toilet itself is actually built from compressed horseshit!

In Norway, meanwhile, poop is already powering buses in the capital of Oslo. The fuel comes from two sewage treatment plants that process the waste of close to a quarter of a million people.

How's it work? No, it's not as if the bus driver is feverishly shoveling shit into a fiery boiler. Instead, when poop is broken down at the sewage treatment plant by bacteria, it creates methane, which can then be used directly to power the bus. The bio-buses cost a little more, but the Norwegians think it's worth the extra scratch. Besides, methane is cheaper than typical gasoline, it's carbon neutral, and it doesn't smell. Or so they tell us. You won't find us sniffing any exhaust pipes in the near future.

KNOW SHIT! ✿

One year's worth of poop from one person can be turned into 2.1 gallons of usable diesel. (We're guessing this number would change according to personal diet, and that a devoted lover of chili-cheese fries may able to provide a little more fuel.)

Eighty buses are already using the poop-based methane, but if the project works out, all of Oslo's four hundred buses will be methane-powered, which could reduce carbon emissions by 30,000 tons each year. Sweden and France are using bio-buses, too. Could our anal output get us around town? That day might not be far off.

Trend 6: Eating Our Poop (Well, Sort Of)

If you don't care to get wattage from your waste, how about getting some roughage instead? That's what's going on in Massachusetts, where the Water Resources Authority takes the shit from forty-three-communities and puts it in people's yards—with a step or two in between, mind you.

In the old days, sludge and scum from Boston's Nut Island sewage treatment plant was pumped into the middle of

Boston Harbor. Then this unholy mix was pumped out with the tide, providing what must have been memorable moments for inattentive yachters. Today that's all changed, as the sludge is converted to Massachusetts's very own Bay Street Fertilizer. Here's how the magic happens. First, sludge is treated as per usual, but then it's dried at high temperatures to toast any remaining bacteria, processed into pellets, and tested to make sure it meets the EPA standards. The end result? Fertilizer that any tomato would love!

Overseas, meanwhile, a product called the Peepoo bag is providing a place to poo where there was none—and providing fertilizer, too. Developed by Swedish researchers, the Peepoo is a single-use biodegradable bag into which goes—you guessed it!—both pee and poo. But like your mom always told you, it's what on the inside that matters. And the innards of the Peepoo bag are lined with a thin film of urea. Once used and sealed, the urea in the bag breaks down the pathogens in the poop and helps to sanitize the waste. The process can take up to four weeks, but then . . . voilà! Some homemade fertilizer.

Trend 7: Drinking Our Poop (Well, Sort Of)

But what if you can't compost, and using a Peepoo bag every day isn't your idea of waste management? For the rest of us, in the years to come, we might just find ourselves drinking

from our toilet, thanks to what's known, rather unappetiz-
ingly, as a toilet-to-tap system.

Nowhere is the trend farther along than in California,
Florida, and Texas, where H_2O is in very short supply. In
Orange County, California, they've wisely opted to call
their conversion project the Groundwater Replenishment
System, instead of toilet-to-tap.

DEEP SHIT!

**Here's a surprise: What's happening in Southern California is old
news in Windhoek, Namibia. Situated in one of the most arid locations in Africa, Windhoek is the first city in the world to re-
claim domestic sewage for drinking water. Built all the way back
in 1967, the Goreangab Water Reclamation Plant supplements
the meager natural water supply.**

Here's how it works. In the past, all treated water went
into the Pacific Ocean, where, unsurprisingly, it quickly
went from freshwater to saltwater. Instead, 70 million gallons a day now go through a treatment process that involves
microfiltration, reverse osmosis, ultraviolet light, hydrogen peroxide, and possibly a written exam. Once mightily
purified, Orange County's water is then piped out to basins
from which it seeps into the ground. The process is so

thorough it supposedly *improves* the quality of the existing groundwater.

Additionally, it will help protect the area against droughts and the necessity of drawing water from other areas. Other cities are considering similar systems. In the meantime, when the next drought rolls around, head to Orange County and look for the water that's clearer than Perrier, bubbling out of the pipe labeled outflow.

Of course, if we're all going to be drinking our poop water someday, somebody better start doing the PR job. After all, who wants to drink the water that came from his toilet—or worse yet, somebody *else's* toilet? One way politicians are tackling the challenge? Showing us that pee-drinking is already happening in much less appealing ways. Southern California, for example, gets part of its water supply from the Colorado River. A number of cities upstream on the Colorado discharge their treated sewage water into the river, including all 2 million residents of Las Vegas. So as the Los Angeles County Economic Development Corporation summed it up, "What happens in Vegas doesn't stay in Vegas."

You Are in Deep Shit— Right Now

Despite all those efforts to move our shit away from us, it turns out that our shit is in fact everywhere. At least, that's the finding of Dr. Elmer Pfefferkorn, a retired professor of virology and parasitology at Dartmouth College. Dr. Pfefferkorn believes that you are currently standing in shit—at least a little of it. According to his theory of a fecal veneer, the world is covered with a microscopic layer of poop.

KNOW SHIT!

Harvard Professor Hans Zinsser agrees with Dr. Pfefferkorn. He once told Pfefferkron that if urine left bright yellow stains and poop bright blue ones, the entire world would be colored bright green.

Pfefferkorn's point is that shit particles pervade the planet. A thin veneer covers everything in your bathroom, most everything everywhere else, and especially electrically charged surfaces like, well, your computer monitor. Says Pfefferkorn, "The fecal veneer is the theoretical construct that the world is covered with a thin layer of feces. You can't see fecal veneer. You can't smell it. But it's there."

The Problem with Being Clean

These days, though, the sanitary revolution—from indoor plumbing to frequent hand washing and sanitizing—has thinned the world's fecal layer. We're literally running out of shit. There is a bit of good news: You're less likely to get certain diseases, like salmonella. And the incidence of parasites such as giardia and the bug that causes amoebic dysentery is lower.

KNOW SHIT!

The first polio epidemic in the twentieth century was in über-clean Sweden—and many researchers believe a too-thin fecal veneer was to blame. In contrast, 98 percent of the population in India is immune to hepatitis A, thanks to a thick fecal veneer.

But overall, the loss of our fecal veneer spells trouble. For example, infants living around a thick fecal veneer respond with the antibodies they've acquired from their moms and quickly develop immunities to a variety of diseases. Later in life, that exposure gives them protection against all kinds of nasty, life-threatening bugs from hepatitis to polio.

All in the Family

One way or another, through the centuries, we've worked awfully hard to get our shit *away.* We've burned it, buried it, and flushed it down rivers. We've tried to make ourselves civilized by distancing ourselves from our very waste, ignoring what is naturally present, yet determined to keep it socially absent. But, like a houseguest who overstays his welcome, our shit just doesn't want to take a hint. And that might not be such a bad thing, after all. In the words of François Rabelais, Renaissance humanist, "O what lovely fecal matter!"

We can all come to realize that our poop is really like a member of our family. We need to be close because we rely on a little poop to get us through life. But spend too much time in each other's company and you'll start to feel a little, well, *nauseated.* At first glance, poop in its humble original form is not much more than filth. But get to know it a little bit, and poop becomes recognizable as a substance of value, whether as compostable night soil or as a late seventeenth-century remedy for the common cold. So no matter what the future brings, from artificial stomachs to toilets that post a note to Twitter when we poop, here's hoping we never stray too far from our shit.

Acknowledgments

The authors wish to gratefully acknowledge the support of the following people who assisted them in getting their shit together: Bob Behrendsen, Elizabeth Beier, Doug Berman, the Blake Memorial Library, Boise, Matt Bowman, John Burke, Laura Colbert, Michele Cormier, Carl Demrow, Dr. John Dunn, Catherine Fenollosa, Elizabeth Field, Janice Gavan, Carol Gregory, Yvonne Jenkins, U.S. space shuttle commander Captain Mark Kelly, Ken Linge, Jamie Maddock, Tom and Ray Magliozzi, Andy Mayer, Don Mayer, Rebecca Oreskes, Dr. Elmer Pfefferkorn, Malcolm Pittman, the Randolph Public Library, Leane Rexford, Rick Sayles, Ben Schott, Al Sochard, Alisa Steck, Roz Stever, Allison Stori, Laura Waterman, Rick Wilcox, Shay Zeller, and William Reed Lamoreux for the generous offer of his meconium.

Bibliography

Books

Diamond, Jared. *Guns, Germs, and Steel.* New York: W.W. Norton, 1997.

George, Rose. *The Big Necessity: The Unmentionable World of Human Waste and Why It Matters.* New York: Metropolitan Books, 2008.

Gregory, Morna, and Sian James. *Toilets of the World.* London: Merrell Publishers, 2009.

Hobson, Barry. *Latrinae et Foricae: Toilets in the Roman World.* London: Gerald Duckworth, 2009.

Kira, Alexander. *The Bathroom.* London: Viking Penguin, 1976.

Lambton, Lucinda. *Temples of Convenience and Chambers of Delight.* London: Pavilion Books, 1995.

Laporte, Dominique. *History of Shit.* Cambridge, Mass.: MIT Press, 2002.

Morrison, Susan Signe. *Excrement in the Late Middle Ages: Sacred Filth and Chaucer's Fecopoetics.* New York: Palgrave Macmillan, 2008.

Veyne, Paul, ed. *A History of Private Life, Volume I: From Pagan Rome to Byzantium.* Cambridge, Mass.: Belknap Press, 1987.

Other Sources

Bloom, Stephen G. "Dr. Fart Speaks." *Salon*, February 24, 2000. www .salon.com/health/feature/2000/02/24/farts

Farivar, Cyrus. "Human Feces Powers Rwandan Prison." *Wired*, July 16, 2005. www.wired.com/science/planetearth/news/2005/07/68127

Yeboah, Kwesi. "Of Underdevelopment and Human Excrement."
   Modern Ghana, March 24, 2003. www.modernghana.com/news/
   111911/1/of-underdevelopment-and-human-excrement.html

Websites

American Restroom Association
   americanrestroom.org/index.html#idx
The Dung File (website focusing on coprolites)
   www.scirpus.ca/dung/human.htm
Facts on Farts
   www.heptune.com/farts.html
Outhouses of America Tour
   www.jldr.com/ohindex.shtml
The Poop Report
   www.poopreport.com
Smelly Poop
   www.smellypoop.com
Sulabh International Museum of Toilets
   www.sulabhtoiletmuseum.org/pg01.htm
Thomas Crapper History
   www.thomas-crapper.com/history02.asp
World Toilet Organization
   worldtoilet.org/index.asp